Praise for *Beauty*

Whether you are a superm⟋ ⟍ , we all
want to be beautiful. In ⟍ ⟍ way, Shelly
Ballestero helps women ackno ⟍ ⟍at we all deal with
inside ourselves and that true be. ⟍ⅉination of mind, body and
spirit. *Beauty by God* offers useful ⟍ ⟍n and beauty tips to pamper your
body and soul—plus interesting facts and information about the beauty
industry we all should know.

—KIM ALEXIS
Supermodel

Your life and beauty issues have just been simplified! No longer must you
choose between healthy or harmful cosmetics or inner or outer beauty . . .
you can have it all! *Beauty by God* is an amazing compilation of spiritual
insight and practical hands-on advice. It is time God's daughters walked
in all the beauty, health and strength He has for them.

—LISA BEVERE
Speaker and Bestselling Author, *Fight Like a Girl*
and *Kissed the Girls and Made Them Cry*

In *Beauty by God,* Shelly takes us on a fantastic journey that bridges our
spiritual walk with God with the outward blessings of living a healthier lifestyle. This book is a must-read for every woman who seeks to
grow deeper in her faith and learn practical tips to look and feel her
very best.

—CANDACE CAMERON-BURE
Former *Full House* Star

Shelly Ballestero embodies beauty from the inside out, and she will inspire you to do the same. In *Beauty by God,* her positive perspective, experience and extensive research combine to give you the motivation and
tools you need to look and feel your very best!

—TAMARA LOWE
Cofounder and Executive Vice President, Get Motivated Business
Seminars, Inc.; Author, *GET MOTIVATED: Overcome Any Obstacle,*
*Achieve Any Goal and Accelerate Your Success*

*Beauty by God* is a great book for women that encourages them not only to be beautiful on the inside but also on the outside. Our bodies are the temple of the living God, and we need to do our best to take care of what the Lord has given us. This book is jam-packed with godly ways of thinking and useful tips and will truly inspire us to be all that we can, spirit, soul *and* body!

—SHANNON NIQUETTE RATLIFF
Christian Author and Runner-up on *America's Next Top Model*

*Beauty by God* is a valuable resource for anyone who seeks to know and understand God's plan for complete health and beauty. Shelly's knowledge and understanding of God's Word will motivate even the most hesitant reader. I encourage you to put what Shelly has written into practice. She has done us a profound service by illuminating the path to beauty and balance from a biblical perspective.

—JORDAN RUBIN
Founder and Chairman, Garden of Life
*New York Times* Bestselling Author, *The Maker's Diet*

I loved every page in *Beauty by God*. Every chapter is filled not only with encouragement but also with practical tips on how to live a healthy life. We have an obligation to take care of our body so that we can finish our race strong, and Shelly gives us great help in doing just that. The resources offered in each chapter are worth the cost of the book! This is a *great* book!

—HOLLY WAGNER
Founder, GodChicks
Author, *GodChicks, Daily Steps for GodChicks* and *WarriorChicks*

Being in the public eye means that I need to try and look my best. So why do I feel guilty when I spend time on myself? *Beauty by God* helped me to see that it is okay to take care of the outside as well as the inside. *Beauty by God* is a handbook for us girls—what a wealth of information! I'm keeping it close by.

JACI VELASQUEZ
Grammy-nominated Recording Artist

# Beauty by God

## Inside-Out Secrets for Every Woman

Shelly
Ballestero

**Regal**

**From Gospel Light**
**Ventura, California, U.S.A.**

Published by Regal
From Gospel Light
Ventura, California, U.S.A.
*www.regalbooks.com*
Printed in the U.S.A.

**Caution:** The information contained in this book is intended to be solely for informational and educational purposes. Some of the products listed in *Beauty by God* are not regulated by the FDA and are used at the consumer's risk. It is assumed that readers will consult a medical or health professional before using any products referred to in this book. The author and the publisher cannot be held responsible for any injury resulting from the recommendations herein, and do not necessarily endorse the products mentioned in this book.

Library of Congress Cataloging-in-Publication Data
Ballestero, Shelly.
Beauty by God : inside-out secrets for every woman / Shelly Ballestero.
p. cm.
Includes bibliographical references.
ISBN 978-0-8307-4684-2 (trade paper)
1. Christian women—Religious life. 2. Beauty, Personal—Religious aspects—Christianity. I. Title.
BV4527.B35 2009
248.8'43—dc22
2008032487

Rights for publishing this book outside the U.S.A. or in non-English languages are administered by
Gospel Light Worldwide, an international not-for-profit ministry. For additional information, please
visit www.glww.org, email info@glww.org, or write to Gospel Light Worldwide, 1957 Eastman
Avenue, Ventura, CA 93003, U.S.A.

*Dear Kelly, I hope you enjoy this Book Love Grandma*

# Contents

*To my grandmother Georgia Jewel Long (d. 2007),*
*who gave me a love for reading.*
*She was the first one to give me a Bible,*
*and I am so thankful she did!*

*To my grandmother Antoinette Benedetto (d. 2006),*
*for her unconditional love.*

*To my mother-in-law, Virginia Ballestero (d. 2006),*
*who believed in me every step of the way.*

*To my mom, Betty Choquette,*
*who has helped me be the person I am*
*through her love and prayers.*
*You are an incredible mother, and I love you!*

*The One who taught me about true beauty—*
*my beloved heavenly Father!*

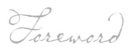

# Foreword

I am so grateful that Shelly Ballestero has stepped out with her message in *Beauty by God*. The truths found in this book will transform every woman from the inside out. For many years, I have seen the inside of the beauty and fashion industry from all angles—the positive and the negative. Though people saw me and still see me as a "supermodel," I truly desire to be a "role model" of a healthy lifestyle.

Unfortunately, the negative messages of today's media have waged a war on the self-esteem of women of all ages. We must begin to stand up and speak the truth: that each woman is created with uniqueness and beauty, inside and out. Shelly, in *Beauty by God*, takes a stand for this truth, encouraging us to begin with a foundation of inner beauty.

I've had a lifelong commitment to athletics, extensive experience in front of the camera, and my own personal encounters with physical trials. These experiences have uniquely informed my understanding of the issues of fitness and women's health, and have challenged me to offer real solutions to women today. In Shelly's book, you'll also find realistic solutions. Her background and education as a licensed esthetician, makeup artist, beauty contributor and herbalist provide the perfect mix to teach us about beauty from the ground up. From great tips on makeup, skincare, hairstyles and clothing—what woman doesn't want that?—to information on skincare product ingredients, toxins and other negative influences on a woman's body, Shelly covers it all. She also teaches us how and why we should be "green" about our skincare and makeup, information that many of us have been missing. Then she digs in to the issues of jealousy and negative thinking that can trap us and keep us from the truth. Finally, Shelly urges us all to live a life of balance and passion.

I hope you'll take the time to read and soak in the message of *Beauty by God*. Shelly Ballestero has truly given us a gift that can ignite the beauty and passion within all women everywhere.

My own personal mission, as a supermodel, role model and spokeswoman, is to combat moral pollution by encouraging people to express true beauty in our superficial age, and to build strong families and healthy lifestyles. Thankfully, Shelly's message has come alongside to help encourage and express the truth to women everywhere. *Beauty by God* will help women discover their true God-given beauty from the inside out.

—Kim Alexis

# Broken Made Beautiful

"If you keep frowning like that, those wrinkles will stay," my mother told me when I was a young girl (I'm Botox-free, so thanks, Mom). My grandmother's advice was, "Stop sucking your thumb or you'll end up looking like Bucky Beaver." (*Is there a beaver named Bucky?* I wondered.)

Other family members teased, "You look like Miss Piggy," or "Look at those thunder thighs!" I knew they were joking, but I took it seriously. Eventually, I assumed the job of criticizing my appearance. I told myself that if my nose were like Elizabeth Taylor's, or if my eyes were blue instead of hazel, or if I were taller . . . *then* I would be beautiful.

I emerged from childhood unable to see my beauty. My view was blocked by my perpetual, negative self-vows that I was not pretty enough. To compensate for my insecurity, I learned at an early age how to use what I did have to manipulate boys to like me. Whether I was beating them at kickball or making them laugh at my celebrity imitations, one way or another I would win.

This need to fight for the attention of men drives many women, no matter what age. Women compare their physical attributes to other females, often viewing them as "competition." Many women have a skewed idea of true beauty that is based on magazines, TV commercials, celebrities or the girl walking down the street with a double-D cup size and long, lean legs. And because men notice, women keep seeking ways to compete in the beauty race. We're all looking for something that will make us stand out, so if it's not our bodies it's our ability to be a top executive, or to drive the newest SUV, or to have the best kids.

I reached the height of my insecurities by selling my self-worth at any cost to be loved. I had my self-confidence literally knocked out of me in an abusive relationship, I did drugs, I tended bar in places where mostly men hung out—and it was all to shut out the negative messages of my past and find a way to feel loved. Soon I realized I was not alone. Most of the females around me in the life I'd chosen—even those I considered beautiful—were unable to see and appreciate their beauty, and they did unthinkable things to feel loved. As sad as it was, being surrounded by people like myself only fed my self-loathing.

It took many years to heal my self-destructive vows so that I could recognize and be grateful for the beauty God has given me. After living so long in the smoke from being so close to the fire (yet not completely burned), I decided I didn't want to live that way anymore. God used a simple thing—a worship music tape called *Shout to the Lord* written by Darlene Zschech, filled with life-giving lyrics—to reach my broken heart. I wept for hours listening to those life-changing words of hope and comfort. Through those songs, God began to turn my heart toward Him.

As I drew closer to God and read what He says about the way He created us and about real beauty, I finally realized that true beauty is a joyful state that can radiate in all of us—through relationships, passion, prayer and, yes . . . brokenness.

As a society, our relationship with beauty is in crisis. We are told that beauty exists only in magazines and within certain age brackets. The media is at war against the average and ordinary, and it assaults us daily with images of how we are supposed to look. Designers are the fashion KGB, brainwashing us on what's "in" this week. This onslaught of media messages leads us to seek out plastic surgery, shopping, anorexia, and bulimia, or chemicals to make us look younger and feel better. Sadly, our culture's obsession with an ungodly view of beauty has blinded us to the beauty in wisdom, nature and, most of all, our spiritual growth.

There will always be someone prettier, someone with better cheekbones or bigger breasts, but what is the endgame in the search for external, fleeting beauty? In the end, no one wins.

A woman's first line of defense in this war for beauty must be against Satan's lies, which cannot nourish or protect us. If we gain control of our thoughts and replace negativity with God's truth, we will find freedom—freedom from fear, freedom from lies and freedom from self.

We want to be physically attractive (and God created us with individual physical beauty), but God wants us to be more concerned with our heart, where our inner beauty arises and shines out because of His love.

Now, girls, I am not saying that you should throw out the hair color and makeup and wear overalls . . . when we look our best, we honor the bodies God gave us. (God's Word speaks of beauty in the Song of Songs and in the story of Queen Esther, who was a Hebrew taken into the "beauty school" of the king's palace. Her physical beauty brought her an audience with the king, through which God saved the Israelites from death.) Nothing is wrong with enhancing our God-given physical attributes, as long as our hearts are pure. What we need is *balance*. Looking our best brings honor to God when our inner beauty is also in balance.

*Beauty by God* offers lots of beauty tips and advice from celebrities, along with fashion guidelines and practical tools to help you look your best. But in these pages you will also make spiritual discoveries and insights to keep your understanding of true beauty real.

> *The king is enthralled by your beauty; honor him, for he is your Lord.*
> PSALM 45:11

## TAKING CARE OF WHAT YOU HAVE

Although the vast majority of us are born with similar physical features on a large scale (head, torso, limbs, and so on), we also are created with a God-given uniqueness and distinctive characteristics that help define us as individuals. Unfortunately, because of the pervasive worldly view of beauty, we often see uniqueness as a flaw. Stop looking for the worst in the mirror and instead see yourself through God's eyes, as one of His beloved daughters. Begin to take care of what *He's* given you, to bring out your inner beauty and shine His love to those around you.

## Your Skin Is the Largest Organ

With that being said, beauty begins with the basics.

My friend Charlotte Hale wrote a book called *The Super Years*, in which she interviewed a beautiful woman named Abbie Busbee, who was the ripe age of 101. Abbie's skin looked virtually unlined, and Charlotte demanded to know her secret. Abbie's magic ingredient was castor oil; she rubbed it on her face and the tops of her hands every night.

Then Charlotte asked her, "Anything you'd do differently if you could go back?"

"Yes, indeed," came the instantaneous reply. "I'd take better care of my teeth. I didn't dream I'd live this long, and I had to get dentures at age 87."

What a hoot Abbie was. We all can learn from women with experience in life. Their wisdom is our gain; the future is a day away and we should treat our temple with care. Personal hygiene is as important to our health as eating right, exercise and avoiding cigarettes and alcohol.

Personal beauty begins with taking care of your largest organ, your skin. Fight the *internal* war on wrinkles so they don't appear externally. In order to restore your skin back to health and give it that radiant glow, it's time to make some changes.

No other organ is so intimately connected to our appearance and our beauty as our skin. Emotions wear on our skin; the environment wears on our skin. When we damage it by self-destructive eating behaviors or negative self-talk, we depreciate our beauty and belittle ourselves.

It is essential to begin healing the skin from within, starting with the least expensive vital beauty regimen: Drink plenty of water! In addition, drink herbal teas, take vitamins and essential oils such as Omega 3s, exercise, pray, and eat organic (when possible) and raw foods.

## Aging Is Inevitable

We have no choice but to age as long as we are living. But we can choose to decide *how* to age (I suggest aging gratefully). The longer we care for ourselves well, the more we can be used for God's purposes. To age well, we must become more conscious of our eating choices, of what we put on our skin, and of how we care for our temple (see 1 Cor. 6:19). We can gain knowledge about beauty products, learn to find economical methods of skin and hair care, and learn to be stylish while preserving modesty. All of this knowledge, combined with God's wisdom throughout the ages, can give you true, godly beauty at any age. Aging is a privilege—I am happy to be here on this planet, living life to the fullest with my family. I am honored to be a wife, mother and a daughter of the King!!

# NATURAL BEAUTY

All of us want to be beautiful, whether we admit it or not. Still, we allow Judge Beauty to sit on our shoulder while we look in the mirror and listen to her say, "Your nose is too big" or "Your arms are too fat for that shirt." Our negative self-talk is a battle that can be won with the weapons God has given us.

God rejoices over His children, so when we put ourselves down, we are disrespecting His handiwork. We cannot allow Satan's lies to gain footing in our minds. We battle back when we replace our self-pity and pride with truth. Matthew 12:34 says, "Out of the overflow of the heart the mouth speaks." What our hearts believe on the inside will come out, not only in our speech but on our faces. What does your heart truly believe about yourself, about what you see in the mirror? You can learn to believe what God knows about you, and then you can learn to allow that inner peace to affect what people see on the outside. And believe me, it will show!

Some of you will flip through this book to see what topics inspire or interest you most, while some will read it cover to cover. Either approach is just fine; there is no wrong way to begin! Whatever way you choose to make the journey, remember that making even small changes in your lifestyle will affect you and everyone around you for the better. There are a *lot* of tips, suggestions and product recommendations in *Beauty by God*, and I don't want you to be intimidated! The important thing is to start somewhere. You don't have to throw everything away in your house, start composting, buy an electric car and become a "green fascist" tomorrow. Simple changes made in gradual steps will lead you to a healthier, more holistic lifestyle.

To take those gradual steps in good company, start a BBG Girl's Club. You and your girlfriends can get together to discuss new products you love, to share great recipes and techniques, and to encourage each other to live up to your God-given beauty. You can even work through this book together! To find out more about BBG Girl's Clubs, go to my website, www.shellyballestero.com.

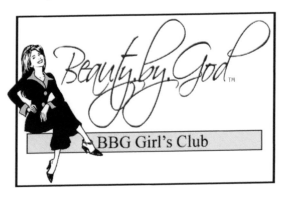

In the following pages, join me as we seek ways to rediscover our natural beauty, both inside and out. Natural beauty consists of a healthy mind, love, peace, charisma, a captivating spirit, healthy cosmetics and the best makeup of all . . . *joy.*

I hope you will find that joy as we explore ways to recapture our *Beauty by God.*

# One

# God's View of Beauty and Balance

Hit the mall . . . turn on the TV . . . open a magazine . . . the world is telling you that beautiful people have it all and that those who aren't so beautiful should feel inferior because they don't. Is it any surprise that the industry responsible for feeding your insecurities through advertisements also sells the "miracle beauty in a jar"?

I personally like the Forrest Gump beauty philosophy: *Beauty is as beauty does.* But how many people really believe that beauty comes from the inside? Not many, if they believe the images perpetually bombarding us at every turn.

No one can keep up with the world's view of beauty; it's impossible. The world's beauty is flawed and, in most cases, unnatural and completely manufactured, manipulated through photographic lighting, computer enhancement and film techniques.

Beauty should be simple, not forced—and it lies within all of us. True beauty comes from our creation by a loving God and our identity in Christ.

Don't you think it's time we recapture our true beauty?

To do so, we need ammunition to fight the world's lies about our lack of beauty. We need to understand how we are manipulated and how our own human minds absorb the messages from the world around us.

*Did you know....?*

❧ That 67 percent of women withdraw from life-engaging activities because they feel badly about their looks? They refuse to go to a special event, or shopping, or to work out, or even to school or to the doctor. Some even avoid stating their opinions because of the way they feel about their looks.[1]

❧ That 90 percent of the world's women ages 18 to 64 want to change at least one aspect of their physical appearance? Body weight ranks the highest.[2]

While I'm glad someone in the secular media is finally telling the truth about beauty, shouldn't those of us who follow Christ be leaders in speaking this positive message? Instead, we continue to buy magazines, watch celebrities, and continue to absorb the wrong messages about our appearance.

Another recent survey by BodyImage Health.org found that:

❧ 65 to 75 percent of females in America at any given time are on a diet of some type.

❧ 75 percent of adolescent girls feel bad about their bodies and 70 percent feel "fat."[3]

Though we may know that God has created each of us with true beauty in His eyes, we are vulnerable to the images that fill our every waking moment.

So what happened? How did our view get so skewed away from the truth?

We complain about beauty and health, yet we continue to idealize our perception of beauty. We think only supermodels and actresses are truly beautiful. We look at their faces and bodies on glossy pages or on the screen and wish that we could look just like that. Then maybe we'd feel good about ourselves.

The reality is, those images we idealize are just that: *ideal,* not real. These women's faces and bodies are made over, touched up and electronically altered to achieve "beauty." The Dove campaign's website includes a video of model Jodie Kidd's face being manipulated right before your eyes. First the makeup and hair, then with the magic touch of Photoshop, her neck becomes smaller and elongated, her eyes are lifted from the brow up, and both sides of her face are slimmed. The final result isn't Jodie Kidd; it's a computerized picture of artificial "beauty" created for the sake of a billboard selling cosmetics. No wonder we have a distorted image of beauty; even our models aren't beautiful enough without "help."

Obviously, our culture's standard of beauty is too high for most women to achieve. It's easy to see why 90 percent of us don't like some aspect of our appearance. While for the majority of women, weight is their number one body-image complaint, even those who don't struggle with weight have something to hate when they look in the mirror.

When I was 10 years old, the thing I disliked most was my hair. I remember wanting to change it, so I got a perm on my already wavy hair. Imagine the outcome! When fifth grade started after the long summer break, there I was: Shirley Temple in the flesh, on the playground ready to play kickball.

Billy was the captain of my team (I was chosen last). My turn came to step up to plate and kick, but then something happened. I looked out at the field and . . . no ball. I heard laughing in the background. *Oops . . . I missed the ball. Didn't even see it.* Billy yelled at me in front of everyone: "Shelly Belly got an ugly perm, and now she can't even kick the ball. I guess those curls took part of your brain! Ha-ha."

I wanted to kick that ball right where Billy . . .

Instead, I ran to the side of the brick schoolhouse and cried my eyes out. I was humiliated.

It was my first encounter with a harsh reality: The way I looked did not measure up to the standards of others. That realization changed my self-image for many years.

Unfortunately, our view of ourselves often doesn't come from how God views us, as it should. Instead, our view of ourselves is often colored by others' opinions, whether warranted or not (usually not). People can be cruel and shallow about how they see others, particularly the opposite sex. Do you remember the movie *Shallow Hal?* The film's reviews weren't that great, but the concept was so true about how men view women. In one of the movie's more memorable exchanges, Tony Robbins is in the elevator with Hal, played by Jack Black, and they are discussing beauty. Hal says he's picky and then explains his desire for the model Paulina, who posed in a *Sports Illustrated* layout.

Tony asks, "You're looking for a young Paulina type?"

Hal responds, "Well, that face, but with better headlights. You know how hers have kind of dimmed lately? Heidi Klum's beams would do. And her teeth. Or, ooh, that Britney Spears girl. She's got great knockers. But she's a tad muscular . . ."

Okay, okay . . . there's more, but you get the picture. Toward the end of the conversation, Tony says, "Okay, Hal, hypothetical situation: Which do you prefer, a girlfriend missing one breast or half a brain?"

"Hmmm, toughie," says Hal. "What about the remaining breast? Is it big?"

Tony gets more than a little frustrated with Hal's shallowness, and he calls Hal on his pattern of judging women by their appearance. He asks Hal if he has ever looked at a woman and thought that he was better than her. Hal answers, "All the time."

Tony puts his hands on Hal's head and yells, "Devils, come out!"[4]

This crude conversation might make us cringe, but it's a humorous snapshot of how many people really view women. And they are not helped by our entertainment industry, which often makes a laughing-stock of women's appearance and self-esteem in order to make more money. Something has gone very wrong. God's view of the beauty within each of us—His creations—is missing from our world, our culture.

What a standard we have to live up to—*Sports Illustrated* models, movie stars, every magazine and TV ad. And now, to make it worse . . . *makeovers*. Now we have to watch "ordinary" people like us transform into perfect versions of their former selves. What was once an unattainable dream—perfect beauty—is now possible if you have the right connections, the right amount of money or the dumb luck to be chosen for a reality TV show. It used

*Did you know....?*

❊ That looking at fashion magazines for just 3 minutes lowers the self-esteem of over 80 percent of women, says Dr. Susie Orbach, a leading British psychotherapist?[7]

❊ That the body fat of models and actresses portrayed in the media is at least 50 percent less than that of healthy women?[8]

to be that a new haircut, a wardrobe change, a visit to the gym or some new makeup would make a women feel great. Now we have television programming like *The Swan, Extreme Makeover* and *Nip/Tuck* to keep us warm and cozy at night with sweet dreams of a cosmetic surgeon re-shaping our worn-out bodies.

Now *that's* entertainment.

We've lost respect for the wisdom that comes with a long life. Aging bodies have become a liability in our culture. Everyone is always looking for the youngest, the freshest, the newest. And as the years wear on, we begin to feel as if we're on the way out the door. Remember the Disney movie *Robots*? Older model robots that become obsolete are remodeled with new and improved shiny shells. In a similar way, women today feel as if they have to keep buying newer, shinier "shells" to be accepted. It's as if the fashion and beauty industry has established a totalitarianism: They decide what's in and what's out (and you're out at 40 years old). What's that about? Haven't they heard that 40 is the new 30? They must not have gotten that memo. (*Note to self*: Rewrite the memo. And this time, click "Send"!)

According to a 1997 Body Shop International campaign, there are 3 billion women who don't look like supermodels and 8 who do.[5] In essence, the whole fashion-and-beauty industry is geared to 8 women. As unrealistic as we know these images to be, we still seek out the newest and best products to make us look more "perfect."

What kinds of companies benefit from making us think our bodies are imperfect? Film and television companies, magazines, diet and cosmetics industries, cosmetic surgeons, fitness gyms, and even the company that produces Barbie dolls. (Speaking of Barbie, have you ever thought about those measurements? Barbie's waistline is the same diameter as her head—wow! Her neck is twice as long as an average human's and her legs are 50 percent longer than her arms. What a role model![6]) Yet even as many of us recognize how we are being manipulated, our self-image still suffers when we compare ourselves to the unrealistic view of beauty portrayed all around us.

In order to stave off the dreaded aging process, and achieve the beauty that culture demands, we've gone from buying makeup to buying new bodies.

Women (and men) now spend countless dollars paying to look younger, thinner, more "beautiful." Procedures now border on an almost-laughable extreme. One can now have an autologous fat transfer, in which a dermatologist withdraws fat from a woman's buttocks and then freezes that fat until her next appointment, when that same fat is injected into her nasal folds or cheeks. (What's next? A famous star auctions off her fat to the highest bidder? I can see the reality show now: *Where the Fat Goes*. Maybe cosmetic surgeons will have their own category at the Academy Awards: "And the Oscar for best surgeon in a drama, for nipping and tucking on Susie Superstar for her role in *Absolute Unreality*, goes to . . ." And the crowd goes wild, because they are all patients!)

> *Did you know. . . ?*
>
> ❄ That in 2005, $15 billion was spent on cosmetic surgery?[9]

This cosmetic surgery industry is raking in the bucks, from tummy tucks to toe tucks. Yes, you heard me right—toe tucks! There is now a procedure called a foot facelift, which is done all for the sake of wearing a $650 pair of Jimmy Choo high heels. Dr. Zong, a Manhattan podiatrist, shortens long toes, smoothes bumpy toes and straightens crooked toes, and he tells his patients, "I'm in the business of 'saving soles.'"[10] Dr. Levine, also of Manhattan, gives foot facelifts too. Some of her other procedures are foot facials, which include salt scrub, mask, peel and massage. (Makes me want to go get one right now!) Some patients undergo injections filled with restylane to cushion their soles from the blow of walking around all day in high heels.[11] One model came into Dr. Levine's office and had liposuction performed on her big toe! (I don't know why we'd be surprised at this; until about 70 years ago, Chinese girls often had their feet bound to keep them small, as tiny feet were a sign of feminine beauty in that culture. Then, as now, what was designed for beauty often became crippling and disfiguring.)

Aside from the fact that cosmetic surgery is often about our misguided attempts to prolong youth and beauty, these procedures also have a deadly side. I read about a woman from Ireland, Kay Cregan, who came to America to have a nose job and facelift. She'd heard about a Dr. Sachs, who gave an acquaintance of Kay's a free facelift in order to drum up business in Ireland. Apparently he had been in more than 30 malpractice suits since 1995, but Kay didn't know that; she just wanted a younger look. Instead, Kay died. The 42-year-old mother of two and wife of Liam suffered "therapeutic complications as a result of the surgery" on March 15, 2005, and was pronounced brain-dead on March 17.[12]

Unfortunately, Kay's story isn't unusual. People die from unnecessary cosmetic surgery.

I had my own scare in this area. In my 20s, I was a bit backslidden in my relationship with Christ (a landslide was more like it). I depended on people around me for my feelings of self-esteem instead of believing in the unique beauty God created in me. I listened much too closely to the words of my abusive boyfriend at the time, who often gave me backhanded compliments, comparing me to his ex-girlfriends. For example: "Shelly, you're not like the women I dated who were models." (He often told me about "the models," even showing me pictures to remind me what they looked like . . . *how kind.*) "They were beautiful and boring, but *you* . . . you're so funny, and have such a great personality, and you're so cute." *Oh, thanks,* I thought. *I'm cute. Like a puppy.*

Needless to say, it's not fun to be compared to other women with better assets—boring or not. And these feelings stayed with me after the boyfriend was gone. Even after I'd met Angelo, who is now my husband, I didn't feel pretty enough. It was like I was still missing the kickball in fifth grade, only now I was missing out on being beautiful. I wanted a nose like Elizabeth Taylor's; I wanted to be taller (couldn't God have given me more than five-feet-four?); I wanted blonde hair and blue eyes (mine were brown and hazel).

So, in my mid-20s, I decided to see a cosmetic surgeon. I told the doctor I wanted Elizabeth's nose. I wanted to look great because I was getting married in a few months.

After the surgery, I was bandaged up like a raccoon mummy. As I lay in recovery, the doctor told Angelo, "There were some complications. When we went in, we discovered that part of the inside of her nose was crushed. I had to fix that first, which took longer than expected, and I could only manage to shorten the tip of her nose a bit. I could not give her the shape she wanted." I had gone through all that pain for nothing. In fact, I saw more imperfections after the surgery than before. (Still, it could have been worse. I heard of a model in New York who had a nose job and got an infection, and then part of her nose fell off. She had to wear a prosthetic nose and face unnecessary disfigurement in the mirror every day.)

This negative surgery experience changed how I saw myself and others. I finally reached a point of acceptance. I began to accept my own appearance without a constantly critical eye, and I began to believe in the beauty that comes from finding my worth in Christ, not from how others see me. My confidence level changed, too. I discovered that when you're confident, you carry yourself differently, and you look more beautiful. Confidence— you can learn to wear it well.

The truth is, there will always be someone prettier than you, taller than you, thinner than you, more toned than you . . . someone with better hair, a smaller nose, longer eyelashes, *whatever*. But you have a special blueprint created by God. You are unique. You have your own look, your own personality, your own gifts—all of which work together to make you beautiful in a way that no one else in the whole world is.

Now, I don't want you to think I'm cursing all makeup or telling you not to seek to look your best (far from it!). We can and should enhance our appearance—in fact, part of this book gives you creative, practical and cost-effective ways to look and feel physically attractive. We can and should seek to look our best at any age, but we also need to learn to see ourselves through the eyes of the One who created us. That point of view will give us a different picture, a true picture of beauty.

## THE BIBLE AND BEAUTY

Romans 12:2 says, "Don't let the world squeeze you into its mold" (*Phillips*). Today we have the radio, billboards, magazines, TV, movies and the Internet passively persuading us until, without even being aware of it, we are "squeezed" into the world's mold.

We should be suspicious about the media when we read in 2 Peter 2:1-3, "There will also be false teachers among you, who will secretly introduce destructive heresies, even denying the Master who bought them, bringing swift destruction upon themselves. Many will follow their sensuality, and because of them the way of the truth will be maligned; and in *their greed* they will exploit you with false words" (*NASB*, emphasis added). We often only read this verse as an occurrence within the context of the Church, but because believers are part of society as well, it could easily apply to our everyday world. False teachers (advertisers and "experts") introduce "new" ways of thinking that are destructive. Their motives? Greed. We are warned not to follow such people (even though it's hard when they have those before-and-after pictures).

This verse also warns against the way (the Christian life) becoming distorted because we follow a lifestyle value that is contrary to the beauty God desires.

So let's look at beauty in its original form: Eve, the First Lady on the earth. The Bible describes her as the mother of all the living (see Gen. 3:20). Eve was fashioned by the hand of our Creator; she was fearfully and wonderfully made! Adam was made out of dirt (I mean dust!), while God designed Eve from living flesh and bone. She was the crown and the pinnacle of God's creation; how beautiful she must have been! She was magnificent, untouched, unblemished by any defect. Eve was flawless, and likely captivated Adam with her strength and beauty. How could she be anything else in a curse-free world?

In Genesis 1:31, we read that God saw all that He had made, and declared it *good*. Our Father gave us the gift of beauty in all areas of life. Look out your back door—what do you see? Trees that bring us life and bear fruit for the hungry; flowers for the smallest creatures to thrive on; grass that provides a sweet carpet for our feet; birds that fill the air with melody. How great is our God to design these extravagant blueprints in our world. He is the greatest Architect.

Yet just after God declared His creation good, everything He made was ruined by sin. Eve bit into Satan's lies—and so began the Fall.

Eve was the first woman to make a mistake with the beauty God created within her, but there are many other women in the Bible whose lives can teach us—women who, though they may have made mistakes, had unmistakable beauty in the eyes of God. One biblical woman, a prostitute named Rahab, owned a house nestled right on the famous wall of Jericho. She was held captive by a monstrous society, a wicked city marked for eternal wrath under God's condemnation. Though Rahab had indulged in sin, she became part of history in one of God's greatest military campaigns. God's grace changed the life, career and future of this beautiful woman.

When Joshua sent his two spies to view the land, they went to Rahab's house. What she did next would have been considered aiding and abetting an enemy of Jericho, yet Rahab had heard of Israel's miraculous escape from Pharaoh across the Red Sea and the drowning of the entire Egyptian army. Though she had sold her body to men, she didn't sell out the two spies, which would have cost her life. She hid the two men on the roof when Jericho's soldiers came knocking on her door. Her bravery not only helped the Israelites capture Jericho as part of God's plan; she became one of only a few women named in the genealogy of Christ's lineage. What an amazing transformation of a formerly sinful woman.

I don't want to get into ethics here; I just want to point out how God transformed a woman from a life of bondage. Rahab is a beautiful example of God's redeeming power. This woman received an extravagant gift— an abundance of grace—and she sipped from the saucer where the cup of God's love overflowed. I stand amazed at how much God loves and forgives us, no matter who we are or what we've done. All we have to do is say, "I believe and receive." That's true beauty.

God also used a beauty pageant to rescue His people, when Esther was crowned queen. The Israelite people were under the rule of a foreign king and were facing a secret conspiracy that threatened their existence. In Esther 2:2 we read that the king was looking for the right queen: "Let a search be made for beautiful young virgins for the king." Esther was lovely in form and features and won the heart and favor of the king. Once chosen, Esther received beauty treatments and special foods. "Before a girl's turn came to go in to King Xerxes, she had to complete twelve months of beauty treatments prescribed for the women, six months with oil of myrrh and six with perfumes and cosmetics" (2:12). Esther was being prepared for the king. But she had a secret that her uncle, Mordecai (her adoptive father), swore her never to tell: her nationality.

Esther was beautiful *and* smart, and to top it off, she had an amazing heart for people . . . her Jewish people. She hid her roots, her very identity, from the king. How terrified she must have been to learn of a murderous conspiracy—an order from Haman (the king's right-hand man) to destroy, kill and annihilate all the Jews!

The law of the land required that anyone who approached the king without an invitation would perish unless the king extended his favor by holding out his gold scepter. It was a risk Esther was willing to take in order to plea for her people's lives. Mordecai fasted for Esther for three days and nights at her request, to pray for her protection in what she was about to do.

Esther used her femininity to catch the eye of the king; she stood in the courtyard wearing her royal robe, hoping that he would look her way. He saw her and was pleased with her and held out his gold scepter, thus sparing her life. He asked her, "What is your request? Even up to half the kingdom, it will be given you" (5:3). Esther requested that the king and his advisor Haman attend a banquet. At the party, the king again asked Esther what request he could grant, and to his surprise, she requested another banquet in honor of the king and Haman. The next night, he again asked to grant her request.

This time, Queen Esther revealed Haman's scheme and begged the king to spare her people. Can you see what's happening here? Esther used the gifts God gave her (her beauty and intelligence) and had the courage to risk her own life for her people. God granted her favor and wisdom to carry out a plan that revealed Haman's plan, which got him hung on the gallows he had built to hang Mordecai!

I love that Esther used her beauty for the glory of her people and her God. She was not boastful or greedy; instead, she was humble and merciful. That is *beautiful*!

On the other hand, we also have examples in the Bible of women who used their beauty in negative, deceitful ways. Delilah used her wiles to trick

Samson, cutting his hair to diffuse the strength God had given him. Fortunately, God used her deceit to bring about His purpose. Then there was Jezebel, a heathen princess who married a king of Israel and brought idolatry, deceit and revenge into God's kingdom. She was so cruel that her name has become synonymous with any wicked woman. Jezebel is the first woman mentioned in the Bible who "painted her eyes" and "arranged her hair." And she did so just before she threw a taunt out the window to her husband and was thrown to her death (see 2 Kings 9:30-37).

There are only two other places in the Bible (Jeremiah 4 and Ezekiel 23) where we see mention of cosmetics ("painted eyes"), and both are shorthand for acting like a prostitute, a metaphor God uses to refer to His people turning against Him and embracing idolatry. Add to that the words from Peter and Paul in the New Testament to caution women against excessive ornamentation and to keep their heads covered (1 Pet. 3:3; 1 Tim. 2:9), and perhaps it's understandable that some Christians shun makeup altogether. Commentaries suggest that these cautions were to keep women with more wealth from creating a gulf between themselves and poor women, which would help to keep early Christian churches from dividing into the "haves" and the "have-nots." Yet some people today take these words to an extreme, and admonish all Christian women to refrain not only from makeup but from any jewelry or "ornamentation." In this way, cosmetics are seen as sinful.

When I was researching this topic, I came across some interesting concepts floating around in cyberspace about cosmetics. One article quoted *Encyclopedia Britannica*, 2001, as defining cosmetics as "beauty products nobody needs."[13] I thought, *Speak for yourself!* Another definition from Wikipedia says, "to enhance or protect the beauty."[14] (I like that definition better.) The word "cosmetics" comes from the Greek word *kosmos*, which means "of this world, worldly."[15] Some might conclude from its word origins that makeup (worldliness) is a sin.

I also found mention of an old law (from the 1700s) stating that a man could get an annulment from his wife if he found out that she had worn makeup during their courtship, which altered her appearance.[16] I guess the divorce rate would be over 95 percent if that were the law now!

## PURSUIT OF BALANCE

In the whirl of all these Scriptures, definitions and opinions, the word that comes to my mind is "balance." We need balance in all areas of our lives, to the best of our ability. Applying balance to our concept of beauty means that even if it's okay to keep our outside appearance looking its best, we need to avoid spending too much time on ourselves, allowing "self" to become our god. I admit that I have fallen into the "self" side of beauty, spending too much money on clothes, makeup and toiletries. And then, feeling guilty from my overspending, I took extra time away from my family to return the items I shouldn't have bought in the first place! (Can I get a reluctant witness?) Balancing beauty with humility is an ongoing battle and a constant struggle.

While I was writing this chapter, I attended a teleprompter class to boost my hosting ability. I walked into the class late with confidence: My hair was okay that afternoon, and even though I was wearing no makeup except Chapstick, I had on a cute outfit.

Every other person there—all women—were well-dressed and wearing beautiful makeup around their perfectly white teeth!

I began to feel awkward. When my turn came for the reading, my heart was in my throat and all eyes were on me. I noticed my earlier confidence beginning to fade as I did a slow dive into the pit of self-judgment. In my mind came thoughts like, *You're speaking too fast—slow down. You're showing too much teeth (forgot those Crest Whitestrips again). Your lips are quivering. Your hair looks like Medusa—don't you believe in defrizzing?*

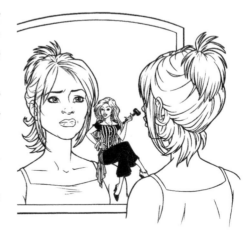

After this beauty battle with myself, I sat back down . . . and so did my nemesis, Judge Beauty, right on my shoulder.

As I watched the playback, the Judge whispered in my ear, *Look at you in that screen—your nose is crooked. Oh, and did you see how one eye is lower than the other? Look at those roots—no, not the movie. Did I mention defrizzing?!* I actually put my book over my face when I saw myself in the monitor, as the casting director critiqued my reading. I think he thought I was nuts!

It's so easy to put ourselves down. When I left the class that evening, I felt degraded by my own ridicule. I could not believe that I had allowed Judge Beauty back in my life, when I knew that she only comes when I invite her. See, we have a higher authority than Old Judge Beauty, and He sits on our other shoulder with the sword of the Spirit in hand, knocking her off with His words of truth! He tells me I am beautiful and captivating and that He delights in me, that He will quiet me with His love, and that He rejoices over me with singing (see Zeph. 3:17).

Our Lord said in John 15:16, "You did not choose me, but I chose you and appointed you to go and bear fruit—fruit that will last. Then the Father will give you whatever you ask in my name." Maybe you asked God to be prettier, to have smaller hips or bigger breasts, or whatever it was that you wanted to change about yourself. You asked and didn't get it. Then you wanted to say . . .

## "GOD SAYS I'M BEAUTIFUL . . . SO WHAT?"

We read in the Bible that God says, "The king is enthralled with your beauty" (Ps. 45:11). We see the beauty in all God has created, and somewhere inside we believe He thinks we're beautiful, but . . .

- A boyfriend or husband left us for a prettier, younger woman.
- We're single (or single again) and have to compete with all those other women out there.
- We know we need to get healthier by losing a few pounds.
- We look at ourselves with a magnifying glass and think others do, too.

Second Corinthians 6:14,17 says, "Do not be bound with unbelievers; for what partnership have righteousness and lawlessness, or what fellowship has light with darkness? . . . 'Therefore, come out from their midst and be separate,' says the Lord" (*NASB*). Paul is talking about not joining in with the crowd. This doesn't have to be a legal thing like marriage or business; it is also true about our *minds*. Don't be bound with the thinking of the dark world around you. Don't let your mind agree with them. They are walking a different path than you are called to walk.

Come out. Be separate. You don't have to become a monk or nun to live intentionally with a value system contrary to the world around you. You don't have to swear off makeup (Lord knows, I love makeup!), because it's a mental battle. *Why are you using makeup? Where do you see your true beauty? If our economy collapsed and you couldn't buy makeup anymore, would you feel ugly all the time?*

> Everything you do, every thought you have, every word you say creates a memory that you will hold in your body.
> —Phylicia Rashad

It is in the mind that the battle rages. The truth is that you must change your perspective. You are beautiful because God made you that way. Beauty is God-encoded deep in your DNA. Now is the time for you to start believing. You are a divinely hand-sculpted masterpiece, fingerprinted body and soul by the most amazing Designer in the universe—none other than our Lord and Savior.

## GREATER IS HE THAT IS IN ME!

Have you ever had your wallet stolen? Suddenly, your personal life is intruded upon; someone knows where you live. It happened to me before, and I was both scared and angry that my identity had been toyed with.

Here is a story about *true* identity theft, beyond what you or I can imagine. This excerpt is from the diary of Lieutenant Colonel Mervin Willett Gonin, who was among the first British soldiers to liberate

Bergen-Belsen in 1945. He is writing about the arrival of a large quantity of lipstick in the days after the camp's liberation.

> I don't know who asked for lipstick. I wish so much that I could discover who did it; it was the action of genius, sheer unadulterated brilliance. I believe nothing did more for these internees than the lipstick. Women lay in bed with no sheets and no nightie but with scarlet red lips; you saw them wandering about with nothing but a blanket over their shoulders, but with scarlet red lips. I saw a woman dead on the postmortem table and clutched in her hand was a piece of lipstick. At last someone had done something to make them individuals again, they were someone, no longer merely the number tattooed on the arm. At last they could take an interest in their appearance. That lipstick started to give them back their humanity.[17]

The Nazis had stripped those beautiful women almost entirely of their identities . . . just as Satan tries to strip us. Sometimes the mask of makeup and clothing is the only shield we have, and making the most of what we've got feels like our only defense. And it's okay. God loves us no matter what we wear. He loves *you*! And He wants to protect you when a harsh, hateful world threatens to undo you.

We are bombarded by messages from the world and by memories from within. Some of our memories are negative words from schoolmates or family regarding our looks, and these are hard to let go of. They can become weapons of an enemy far more evil than Judge Beauty: Satan, whose tactic is to trick us into believing lies. He wants to kill, steal and destroy, and he takes pleasure in shooting all kinds of fiery darts at us, aiming at the bull's eye (our minds). But guess what? We have a superior power. When those darts come a-flyin' . . . dodge, jump and catch! Take them in your hands and destroy them with the words of our Lord: "Satan, get behind me. You have no power over my mind!"

I read an article about a young girl from Haiti, who was an adorable sweet-looking child. The first picture I saw was taken when she was 18 months old. The next picture showed her at 13 years old, with a 21-pound tumor consuming her face. All you could see were her nostrils, her eyes and one tooth. This precious child could not talk because of the growth, so she had invented her own language. After many years of torment (cruel people would stop and scream "Cow" or "Monster" when she walked down the street), all the mirrors had to be taken out of her house because seeing her reflection became even more painful than the name-calling.

After a fruitless search for a doctor to help her, the girl's mother heard on TV about the Haitian nonprofit organization Good Samaritan for a Better Life. She contacted them, and they sent the girl to Florida to remove the tumor. She is now 15 years old, and after three surgeries (with more still to come), she says, "Although my face is still distorted compared with other kids', I don't hide anymore when I see people. I feel beautiful."[18]

Wow! Out of the mouths of babes! The burden this girl had carried for so long was heartbreaking; I was ashamed at how much I care about my looks. How can we put so much emphasis on outward appearance when we see a girl who is dealing with such deformities, radiating such confidence?

I am reminded by stories like hers to look at myself with kinder eyes. Perhaps you've already learned to do that. If not, think back to a time when you were young. Imagine a photo of yourself as a little girl—so innocent, content, filled with optimism and joy.

I think back to a picture of my dad with me on his lap, wearing my white coat and a smile ear to ear—so secure in the love of my dad. So happy; not a care in the world. I was beautiful—my dad told me so. On days when I feel ugly, instead of listening to Judge Beauty's self-condemning verdict or walking away with my head down, I look beyond my reflection and see my younger self—the happy one who is content and beautiful!

Yet even beyond the innocent face of your youth, learn to look deep within to see that you are a daughter of the King. He is enthralled with you. He sings over you. He loves you unconditionally. He knows your true beauty and He wants to remind you of it, too.

*Beauty can be bought by man, but your soul was paid by death.* God sent Jesus to die in order to pay for the ugliness of sin. In His resurrection, He restored the beauty of your relationship with God. The more you let His unconditional love transform you, the more your true beauty will shine from the inside out.

God's love can actually transform your face. When you are content, tiny muscles in your face are relaxed. Have you ever seen a person who has had a hard life, filled with abuse, alcohol, drugs or self-sabotage? Then one day they give their life over to God and their very face is transformed. Peace has taken over; love has entered their life; divine beauty has taken the place of hardness and hardship.

God wants us to accept ourselves just as we are. He loves us and our imperfections. He wants us to be beautiful without the vanity. That is attainable with balance and acceptance of what He has given us and how He created us.

Yes, we can do our best to look our best, as long as we remember that our best should always be intended to give God glory. Real beauty isn't about makeup, the latest trends or the perfect body; it's about looking life right in the face and seeing God's glory.

In *Beauty by God* you will discover helpful tips for making the most of your God-given appearance, for making wise and economic choices about skincare and hair care, for looking your best. Yet above all, remember that your body is God's dwelling place, which is the number-one reason to take care of it to the best of your ability.

> People are like stain-glass windows. They sparkle and shine when the sun is out, but when the darkness sets in, their true beauty is revealed only if there is a light from within.
> —Elisabeth Kübler-Ross

# Beautiful

*Hello my friend I'm wondering how you've been*
*The last time we talked I heard the pain within*
*You really need to know I really need to help you see*
    *(this is your destiny)*
*The miracle you are everything you were born to be*

*You are beautiful*
*A shining star is what you're meant to be*
*You're beautiful*
*A brilliant light for all of the world to see*

*So now my friend you're seeing light come in*
*The truth now revealed this is where life begins*
*You'll never be alone surrounded by a love that's true*
    *(He'll lead you through)*
*So let the road unfold find what He promised you*

*You are beautiful*
*A shining star is what you're meant to be*
*You're beautiful*
*A brilliant light for all of the world to see*

*You are stronger then you realize*
*I can see it in the way you move*
*Stop listening to those lies*
*It's time they see the real you*

*You are beautiful*
*A shining star is what you're meant to be*
*You're beautiful*
*A brilliant light for all of the world to see*

# TWO

# Get Glowing, Gorgeous and Green

You've heard the saying "Beauty is only skin deep," right? But have you heard that beauty actually begins deep on the inside?

Did you know that sugar ages your skin?

That an excessive amount of coffee not only makes your heart beat faster but can also bring on wrinkles earlier?

Did you know that fats and soda (yes, diet soda too!) contribute to the aging factor?

Would you believe me if I told you that you could look 10 years younger without having plastic surgery? Or would you rather hand over your money to the marketing gurus behind the "No More Wrinkle" crème campaigns for the promise of younger-looking skin? Don't get me wrong—some crèmes do offer benefits. But the bottom line is that what you put into your body is reflected on the outside. In fact, beauty goes much deeper that your skin—all the way to your organs.

In this chapter, we look at a multitude of ways to nurture your natural beauty from the inside out. I've got plenty of tips in upcoming chapters for making the most of your outer beauty, but let's start by looking at how you can treat your insides to the same careful attention you pay to your outsides!

# GET GLOWING!

## Drink Your Way to Health

Yes, drinking plain, clear, purified water offers some of the best anti-aging benefits ever. Water is the bedrock of our bodies, making up two-thirds of our total volume, so it only makes sense to supply ourselves with clean, pure $H_2O$. Water hydrates cells, flushes out toxins, helps with digestion, and reduces headaches and dizziness—not to mention helping with weight loss and increasing energy.

In his book *Perfect Weight America*, Jordan Rubin discusses purified water and how it can be overlooked as a weight-loss tool because it is ordinary. "What water does is . . . revs up your metabolism and hydrates the cells so that you can process carbohydrates and fat more efficiently. When your body is well hydrated, you accelerate the liver's ability to convert stored fat into usable energy and help your kidneys flush out toxins. A good rule of thumb is a half-ounce of water for every pound of weight," Rubin recommends.[1]

### Get Purified!

Why purified water? For starters, purified water is safer than tap water because it contains no harmful chemicals. Some water filters even eliminate bacteria, viruses and parasites. Maybe the most tangible benefit of drinking purified water is the great taste. With the impurities and contaminates removed, all that remains is the clean, refreshing taste of pure water. Who knew that a tall, cool glass of water could be a special treat?

### Get a Filter

When traveling, Jordan Rubin uses a portable filtered water system by Aclare, available from www.healthyperceptions.com. The owner of the company, Tim Kerr, and his son, John, are an extraordinary team. In 1987, Tim designed, patented and manufactured the first-ever shower filtration system. His revolutionary design is now used by many other shower filter manufacturers. We have one at home, and we definitely feel the benefits— from having a better hair day to softer skin. The chlorine in shower water has a harsh, drying effect on skin and hair. Also, skin pores widen while you shower, making dermal absorption of chlorine and other chemicals possible. The chlorine can cause rashes and other skin irritations if it is absorbed by the skin.

## Get Rid of Plastic Bottles

As much as possible, keep your water out of plastic bottles. Especially when water bottles have been left in a hot car, the vapors released are toxic. Instead, go for an alternative water bottle made from safe material. Look at your local health food store or try www.siggs.com or Camelbak (can be found at Sports Authority or other outdoor stores). It may set you back a few bucks on the front end, but you can save over a thousand dollars annually by filling your bottle at home with filtered water instead of buying disposable plastic. Plus, it helps save the environment.

## A Good Night's Sleep

People who sleep for eight hours reap a host of health benefits. Ample shut-eye encourages your body to produce more of the "fullness" hormone, called leptin, and less of the "hunger" hormone, ghrelin. Plenty of sleep also helps ease anxiety and depression, which can trigger emotional eating.[2]

# LIFESTYLE AND ENVIRONMENT

## Air Quality

The quality of the air in your home is important to your health. Indoor air at times can be more polluted than outdoor air. Ventilate your home frequently, especially while cleaning. Open the windows to let in clean, fresh air and let out stale, used air. When it's not possible, due to unfriendly weather, to keep outside air flowing in, consider investing in an air purifier or energy recovery ventilator (ERV).[3]

## Replace Cookware

Take a close look at what you cook with. If some of your Teflon-coated pots and pans are scratched, you need to replace them at once. According to the Environmental Working Group (EWG) and the Campaign for Safe Cosmetics (a coalition of health, labor, environmental and consumer-rights groups), the coating on nonstick cookware contains a chemical called polytetrafluoroethylene (PTFE). DuPont's Teflon is the most well-known brand. When heated to very high temperatures, this coating creates hazardous fumes.[4] If you use nonstick pans, be sure to avoid high temperatures; use medium heat and then reduce to a lower temperature. DuPont does not recommend heating Teflon pans higher than 500 degrees. I recommend choosing seasoned cast-iron, non-lead ceramic ware, stainless steal or non-aluminum pans instead.

## Naturally Clean

Many household cleaning products contain toxic chemicals that create an unhealthy environment in your home. Many new nontoxic housecleaning product lines are now available at more budget-friendly prices (see the Resources section for a product list), or you can make your own with vinegar, lemon or baking soda. Toxic ingredients to avoid in your cleaning products include: ammonia, formaldehyde, hydrocarbons or petroleum distillates, chlorine bleach, dyes, glycols, and phosphoric and sulfuric acid.

## Avoid the Microwave

Microwaves have become an integral part of our culture; however, we should be more cautious than we are about their potential hazards. There is some evidence that suggests microwave ovens can leak very small amounts of radiation (especially around the oven door), so it is best to stand at least four feet away while your food is heating up (or avoid using the microwave oven altogether!).

It is best to use a glass container or nonleaded microwavable ceramic when heating your food in a microwave. Avoid using plastic storage containers such as margarine tubs, takeout containers and other one-time use containers in the microwave. Chemicals from the plastic can leech into microwaved foods, and these chemicals (such as DEHA, DEHP, MEHP or PET) can be dangerous to your health. Also, never use thin plastic storage bags, brown paper or plastic grocery bags, newspaper or aluminum foil in the microwave oven. And, to be extra safe, be sure to not let plastic wrap touch foods during microwave cooking (if you choose to use plastic wrap).

## YOU ARE WHAT YOU EAT

Another significant aspect of cultivating beauty from the inside out is what you eat. You can create a nontoxic, clean and beautiful environment, but if you are not eating healthy foods on a regular basis, it will show on the outside—not just in your skin, but in those few unhealthy pounds. Now, I'm not saying you have to be skinny to be healthy or that skinny people are healthy (or, for that matter, that you will be skinny if you eat only healthy food). Our beauty and self-esteem come from God, and have very little to do with our body size. But taking care of the body He gave us includes making healthy choices about what we put into it.

Some of us may need to lose weight to be healthier, but we can't all be a size 2! In fact, like Queen Latifah says on those Jenny Craig commercials, it's not about fitting into a dress size; it's about being a size healthier. If you are unhealthy in your weight, whether too thin or too large, you and your doctor can determine what size you need to be to be healthy. But what's the best way to get there?

### Best-Kept Diet Secrets

One of the best-kept diet secrets is *No diet*. The first three letters in "diet" are D-I-E, and unfortunately there have been more than a few people who have died from extreme dieting measures and weight loss. Our goal is to live life to the fullest, the way God intended . . . and that means staying alive to enjoy the beauty He is growing in us! If you need to lose some weight to get healthy, make sure you take the right approach—a healthy approach. And see your doctor to make sure you consider *all* your health issues before you begin.

I really don't like the fad diets out there. Most of them are heavy on hype, when really all you get are expensive packaged meals filled with preservatives and fillers. Where is the nutrition in that? You don't need that kind of help.

It's truly not as hard as it sounds to eat well, if you follow the first rule of proper nutrition and weight control: plan, plan and plan. You've probably heard the saying, "If you fail to plan, you plan to fail," and this is certainly true with meals. Preparation is key. If I don't start thinking about our family's evening meal the night before (or at least the morning of), we end up eating out . . . which happens more often than I like. Think ahead and make a plan, and you'll have no need of pricey diet gimmicks.

I eat my way to beauty by choosing good fats (omega-3, mono- and polyunsaturated) and good carbs (natural and unrefined) and staying away from sugar during the week. I eat half portions—about the size of my fist—of protein and carbs, and I snack on veggies, fruits and almonds. On the weekend, I make chocolate chip cookies (I love chocolate chip cookies!) or another treat, but I replace the sugar in the recipe with agave nectar, honey or Xylitol. I complete a detoxification program a few times a year, and keep my pantry empty of soda or diet soda, sugary so-called "juice" drinks and anything artificial.

Yes, my kids get upset when they're around other kids. They tell me how deprived they are, but I just smile and tell them they will be glad for their "deprivation" one day. Besides, it's not as if they never get any junk food; they do . . . but the "junk" is made with organic ingredients. They are even allowed one soda per week! (Okay, some of you think I'm nuts. But I know how bad soda is for their health!)

Here are a few other guidelines I try to follow to make the most of what I eat.

## Avoid MSG

Many of us, at one time or another, have had some kind of MSG reaction—from headaches to gaining weight—whether or not we knew the chemical food additive was the cause. The first published report of a reaction to monosodium glutamate appeared in 1968, when Robert Ho Man Kwok, M.D., who had emigrated from China, reported that although he had never experienced the problem in China, about 20 minutes into a meal at certain Chinese restaurants in the U.S., he suffered numbness, tingling and tightness of the chest lasting for approximately two hours. In

1969, John W. Olney, M.D., reported that laboratory animals exposed to monosodium glutamate suffered brain lesions immediately and neuroendocrine disorders later in life.

MSG is found in most soups, salad dressings, processed meats, frozen entrees, ice cream and frozen yogurt; in some crackers, bread and canned tuna; and very often in "low fat" and "no fat" foods to make up for flavor lost when fat is reduced or eliminated. It can also be found in cosmetics, pharmaceuticals and dietary supplements, as well as internal feeding products, infant formulas, vaccines (including those used on children) and IV formulas used in hospitals for very sick patients.[5]

## Not a Sweet Deal

Processed, refined sugar is at the top of the list of what *not* to eat if you're concerned about health and beauty. Not such a sweet deal after all, sugar can make skin dull and contribute to wrinkles by damaging collagen and elastin, the protein fibers that keep skin firm and elastic. When skin is damaged, it is less supple and becomes dry and brittle. Plus, sugar can negatively affect your body's natural antioxidant enzymes, increasing the chance of sun damage—the main source of aging skin.

## Diet Soda Lovers, Watch Out!

In a study conducted by researchers at Purdue University, artificial sweeteners—such as those found in diet soda—increased calorie intake, body fat and weight gain in rats. The study also found that artificial sweeteners may disrupt the body's natural ability to "count" calories based on foods' sweetness, thereby changing your body's ability to regulate calorie consumption. This finding may explain why increasing numbers of people in the United States lack the natural ability to regulate food intake and body weight. According to one of the researchers, associate professor Susan Swithers, "Increased consumption of artificial sweeteners and of high-calorie beverages is not the sole cause of obesity, but it may be a contributing factor. It could become more of a factor as more people turn to artificial sweeteners as a means of weight control and, at the same time, others consume more high-calorie beverages to satisfy their cravings."[6]

Instead of artificially sweetened sodas and fruit drinks, choose teas instead; green, roobias, white, chamomile, mint, holy basil and kombucha teas are healthy and great-tasting options.

## The 100-Calorie Snack Section

Each of these lip-smacking snacks has only 10 calories. Satisfy your hunger by mixing and matching to build your own personalized 100-calorie snack.

| | | |
|---|---|---|
| 1 navel orange segment | 12 blueberries | 2 large strawberries |
| 3 watermelon balls | 1 apple slice | 1 large celery stick |
| 3 cherry tomatoes | 3 green grapes | 2 carrots |
| 20 roasted and salted soy nuts | 1 cashew half | 1 pecan half |
| 4 cheddar Goldfish® crackers | 42 Cheerios® | 3 plain M&Ms® |
| 1/3 cup air-popped popcorn | 7 pieces Pirate's Booty™ | 1 peanut M&M® |

## A Word About Organic

My kitchen pantry and fridge are filled mostly with USDA-certified organic foods; our family has been eating this way for well over a decade. I was at the front door when the first Whole Foods market came to town—40 minutes from my home, but I was first in line (should have gotten a door prize)—several years ago.

During the last 12 years, we have learned a lot about pesticides and food additives, and the more we learn, the more convinced we are that choosing organic over more conventional foods is the healthier option. Organic farming relies on ecologically based practices such as cultural and biological pest management, and excludes all synthetic chemicals, antibiotics and hormones in crop and livestock production.

Learning about organic can be confusing when it comes time to buy it for your kitchen. What does it mean when something is labeled "natural," "organic," "free-range" or "certified organic"? Here are a few terms you'll see on products, along with their definitions:

- *Certified organic*: The product has been produced according to the National Organic Program's (NOP) guidelines and certified as compliant with the rules by an independent, USDA-accredited certifier.

- *Organic, not certified*: The grower or producer has met the NOP guidelines, but sells less than $5,000 per year of the product directly to consumers (not as ingredients to USDA-certified producers). This is usually the case with small, local farmers.

- *Natural*: The product contains no artificial ingredients or added colors and is minimally processed in a way that does not alter the raw product. The label must explain its use of the word *natural*, such as "no artificial flavor or color."

- *Free-range*: Currently, the USDA has only defined free-range standards for poultry (you'll also see it on eggs), but not for beef, pork or other livestock. Free-range chickens and turkeys are not caged and have at least limited access to the outdoors.

- *Grass-fed*: Grass-fed animals (usually beef or milk cows) eat only what they were designed to eat: grass. They are allowed continuous pasture access to graze, rather than being fed grain or grain-based products. Organic regulations do not require grass feeding exclusively.[7]

In their book *A Field Guide to Buying Organic*, Luddene Perry and David Schultz educate readers about raw food preparation, from cultivation (usage of fertilizer and pesticides) to methods of processing. For instance, a label for olive oil may say "cold pressed," but Perry and Schultz explain that the phrase has no legal meaning. They suggest that instead you should look for a label that clearly states that the oil was *refrigerated expeller pressed*, which means that no heat or solvents that might contaminate the oil were used. I recommend Perry and Schultz's book to anyone who wants to become a label-smart, organic-educated consumer.[8]

## Produce
Even when shopping for healthy, raw foods, take care choosing what you put in your shopping cart—especially if you are not buying organic produce.

Check out the foods on the list below from the Environmental Working Group before you buy your produce. (You'll notice that I refer to the excellent research done by the EWG throughout this book. You can sign up to receive updates on their most recent findings at www.ewg.org.) The foods on the left consistently have the highest pesticide count, while those on the right have the least. (A reminder: When you take home your produce, no matter how clean it might seem, be sure to wash well before eating or cooking.)

| Worst | Best |
| --- | --- |
| Peaches | Onions |
| Apples | Avocado |
| Sweet bell peppers | Sweet corn (frozen) |
| Celery | Pineapples |
| Nectarines | Mango |
| Strawberries | Sweet peas (frozen) |
| Cherries | Asparagus |
| Lettuce | Kiwi |
| Grapes (imported) | Bananas |
| Pears | Cabbage |
| Spinach | Broccoli |
| Potatoes | Eggplant [9] |

## Change the Way You See Food

In researching this book, I spoke with Donna Schuller, wife of Crystal Cathedral's senior pastor, Robert Schuller. Donna is a certified nutritional consultant. When we spoke, she and her husband were in the middle of an UltraClear cleanse (by Metagenics), which is designed to detoxify the liver. With any cleanse, there are certain food restrictions, and as we discussed these, Donna commented that people generally focus on what they *can't* eat instead of what they *can* eat. Because of this mindset, people talk themselves out of healthy eating or a cleanse. Donna chooses to focus instead on the benefits: what she *can* eat and the positive results of a little perseverance for her overall wellbeing. Now *that's* a healthy way to look at taking good care of our bodies!!

## SUPPLEMENTAL BEAUTY

Even when we eat well most of the time, the high-stress, high-octane lives most of us lead mean that our bodies need additional help. This is why we need supplements. Many supplements that improve the function of our internal organs can also have anti-aging affects on the external. Lynn Schultz, cofounder of 1-800-HEALTHY says:

> The way we feel about ourselves relates to the appearance of our hair, skin and nails. Accordingly, we tend to give these tissues a great deal of attention once they are on the outside of our body. But we give them very little attention when they are on the inside, actually being grown. We spend a fortune enhancing the outside of our bodies with beauty products—manicures, pedicures, hair color, hair treatments, acrylic nails, porcelain nails, and more. The problem is that by the time we see these tissues, they're technically dead and their health cannot be enhanced, only their appearance can. What makes more sense is to support the healthy growth of these tissues at the only time it can be done—when they are on the inside being created.[10]

Ingredients to look for in anti-aging supplements include organic alfalfa; grapeseed extract; vitamins A, C, E and D; R-lipoic acid; biotin; choline; inositol; calcium, copper, iodine, zinc and phosphorous; hyaluronic acid; gingko biloba; Siberian ginseng; lecithin; antioxidants; protein; fiber; essential fatty acids; food-grade collagen; and green tea. Everyone is different, which means that everyone has different deficiencies that should be supplemented. When it comes to choosing a combination of supplements, getting the proper recommended daily dosage and ensuring that you avoid interactions with other medications, see your physician, chiropractor or naturopath. Ask what brand(s) he or she recommends for potency, purity and accurate labeling.

Fish oil and cod liver oil are also wonderful supplements to consider. Cod liver oil has been used for over 150 years in the U.S. In an interview,

Jordan Rubin told me, "I think fish oil is beneficial, but cod liver oil is so much more important for human health. Cod liver oil has all the omega-3s of fish oil (EPA and DHA) along with the crucial fat-soluble vitamins A and D, which most American's are deficient in."[11] He recommends that anyone using fish oil switch to cod liver oil to support immune function, breast health, bone health, cardiovascular health and a healthy mind. (If you eat vegan, try hempseed or flaxseed—both are great on salads!)

## DETOXIFY FOR HEALTH[12]

Americans are becoming more aware of the importance of eating sensibly, exercising moderately, drinking adequate quantities of clean water, consuming quality supplements and managing their weight. However, there is increasing evidence that stress has created a population of sugarholics. How? Research has shown that stress causes the adrenal glands to release excess cortisol, a stress hormone that triggers overindulgence in simple carbohydrates—chocolate, candy, sodas and ice cream, for instance—even when they are not hungry. The average American adult consumes 3.5 pounds of sugar per week; children consume even more. If the present trend continues, the percentage of overweight American adults will increase from 67 percent to 75 percent by 2015, portending profound effects on individuals, families and even the nation's public health.[13]

Let's take a look at what goes into our bodies daily: processed food, sugar, chemicals such as food preservatives and cleaning supplies, caffeine, smoke (first- or second-hand), diet and regular soda, polluted air, cosmetics, hair and body products, and water. To make matters worse, many of us have parasites. Yes, these harmful creatures lurk around on just about every living thing—humans included—inside and out. Yuck! As these chemicals, toxins and parasites accumulate in the body over time, they can cause the liver and kidneys to become overworked and weak.

With all that consumes us—from toxins to stress—we need to fight back! Here are some ways to diffuse the bomb of chemical warfare with detoxification.

## Cleansing Out the Toxins

Various commercial body cleanses are becoming more popular, but with so many available, how do you know which one is for you? It's tough to choose, especially if you have certain constraints, ranging from a thyroid condition to a heart condition. I suggest a cleansing program with 100-percent natural ingredients (that is, no artificial or genetically modified ingredients). These programs usually consist of supplements and shakes from the program's manufacturer, and determination provided by you. (See the Resources section for recommendations.) Follow directions and recommended daily dosages carefully, and *talk to your doctor before beginning any cleansing or detoxing regimen.*

Instead of using a commercial program, you can detox on your own, using a simple routine like the seasonal cleanse recommended by Jordan Rubin (see below).

### *Seasonal Cleansing*

In traditional Chinese medicine, it is believed that cooked foods have warming properties for the body and raw foods have cooling properties. The challenge is to eat cleansing foods according to what the body needs—warming or cooling. For someone living in Idaho in mid-February, juicing carrots and eating watermelon won't do them much good! Instead, they should consume hearty soups, cooked veggies, lean meats, cooked whole grains and healthy oils.

Jordan Rubin recommends a 10-day cleanse quarterly in January (winter), April (spring), July (summer) and October (fall). In winter, try to eat 75 percent cooked foods and 25 percent raw foods. In spring and fall, eat 50 percent cooked foods and 50 percent raw foods. In summer, eat 25 percent cooked foods and 75 percent raw foods. During each 10-day cleanse, eat every two to three hours, five times a day, from the suggested food list for each season:

**Winter**: beets, cabbage, carrots, citrus fruits, daikon radishes, onions, rutabagas, turnips and winter squash

**Spring**: asparagus, blackberries, green onions, leeks, lettuces, new potatoes, peas, red radishes, rhubarb, spinach, strawberries and watercress

**Summer:** apricots, blueberries, cherries, eggplant, fresh herbs, green beans, hot peppers, melon, okra, peaches, plums, sweet corn, sweet peppers, tomatoes and zucchini

**Fall:** apples, broccoli, Brussels sprouts, cauliflower, collards, grapes, kale, pears, persimmons, pumpkins, winter squash and yams[14]

This recipe, from Jordan's late Grandma Rose, is great for any season. Her tasty soup can be used as a meal during most cleanses . . . or any time!

### Cleansing Chicken Soup[15]

| | | |
|---|---|---|
| 1 whole chicken (free-range, pastured or organic chicken) | 3-4 quarts filtered water | 2-4 tbsp. Celtic sea salt |
| 6 celery stalks | 1 bunch parsley | 2-4 zucchinis chopped |
| 1/2 cup fresh or frozen peas | 4 medium-sized onions, coarsely chopped | 4 inches grated ginger |
| 1 tbsp. raw apple cider vinegar | 5 garlic cloves | 4 tbsp. extra-virgin coconut oil |
| 1 pound green beans | 8 carrots, peeled and coarsely chopped | 1-1/2 tsp. cayenne pepper |

*Remove fat glands and gizzards from the cavity of the chicken. Place chicken in a large stainless steel pot with water, vinegar, garlic, ginger, salt, cayenne pepper, extra-virgin coconut oil and all vegetables except parsley. Let stand for 10 minutes before heating. Bring to a boil, removing the scum that rises to the top. Cover and cook for 8-12 hours. (The more you cook the stock, the more cleansing it will be.) About 15 minutes before finishing the stock, add parsley. (This will impart additional mineral ions to the broth.) Remove from heat and take out the chicken. After it cools, remove chicken meat from the carcass, discarding the bones. Drop the meat back into the soup. You may puree for even easier digestion.*

## Internal Pest Control

Antiparasite support is next in our plan of action, because "every living thing has at least one parasite that lives inside or on it, and many, including humans, have far more."[16] The combination of environmental toxins, unhealthy diet and parasites poses a grave danger to humans. "Parasites have killed more humans than all the wars in history," reported National Geographic in its award-winning documentary *The Body Snatchers*.[17]

Dr. Gloria Gilbére, author of *I Was Poisoned by My Body*, suggests a homeopathic formula called Homeopathic Parasite (find it at www.herb specialists.com), in combination with Zymex 11.[18] Her protocol for the parasite cleanse is two weeks on, one week off, for a period of eight weeks. Then you are finished—and so are those creepy bugs!

## Spring Clean Your Colon

To sweep your colon clean, Dr. Gilbére recommends BioEudaemonic Nutritionals Colon Sweep. She says, "In order to consume sufficient fiber for a clean colon, you would have to eat approximately two large turkey-platter-sized plates of raw vegetables daily—not likely to be accomplished in a typical busy lifestyle. Colon Sweep sweeps away the sludge within the intestinal walls. After all, scientists have confirmed over 80 percent of our immune system is based in our gut!"[19]

Two platters of vegetables a day might not be realistic, but you can help your colon by making this delicious salad.

### Good for Your Colon Salad [20]

1 head cabbage (green or white), shredded or finely chopped
3 grated carrots
1 avocado, sliced

**Dressing:**
2/3 cup flax seed oil
1/4 cup Bragg Liquid Aminos
Dulse flakes, garlic powder, onion powder to taste

*Combine dressing ingredients and mix well, then drizzle over salad ingredients and serve (makes 2 to 4 servings).*

## Take a Probiotic

During my interview with Charlie Skeen, vice president of Product Development Nutrition at Premier Labs, he stressed the importance of taking the right form of minerals your body needs during detoxification, as well as taking an effective probiotic to keep friendly intestinal bacteria intact.

Without good bacteria, our body is unable to digest food properly. Our intestines become overrun with toxins and waste, which restricts the absorption of nutrients and sets the breeding ground for disease. When we frequently ingest chlorinated water, coffee, alcohol and fatty foods, or when we get stressed or overly tired, we unknowingly kill the good bacteria in our bodies. Even the foods we eat to stay healthy—such as meat and milk—contain antibiotics and hormones, which further reduce the levels of good bacteria.

A probiotic encourages the growth and health of good intestinal bacteria. As with all supplements, check with your doctor before you begin taking a probiotic.

## Detox Food Dos and Don'ts

You might wonder what foods you should eat while detoxifying. Well, wonder no more! Organic raw fruits and veggies, legumes, whole grains, nuts and seeds, good fats (especially omega-3), plenty of purified—not tap—water and green tea are the best places to start. (My favorite green tea is by Pure Inventions. I love the quality, and the price is not bad when you consider that one dropper of the concentrate is equivalent to 14 cups—providing more than 80 mg of green tea antioxidants!)

Keep these healthy snacks on hand during your detox to avoid cravings and to realize the maximum cleansing benefit: raw almonds, Lärabar or Gopal's Rawma bar (raw food bars), organic Granny Smith apples or celery with raw almond butter, flaxseed crackers, fruits and veggies.

There are certain foods you should avoid while undergoing a detox, including milk and other dairy products, processed foods, hydrogenated oils and soy protein, pork, high fructose corn syrup, sugar, white flour products, artificial sweeteners, soft drinks, tap water, margarine, black tea and coffee (try a coffee alternative such as Teeccino or Cafix).

## Detox Blues

As your body cleanses itself, you may experience headaches, nausea and/or fatigue, because the toxins are leaving your body. Everyone is different; while one person may experience minor symptoms, others may experience more dramatic effects. Get plenty of rest and go to bed early, which will also help fight food cravings. Stay hydrated by drinking plenty of purified water, especially if you feel a headache coming on.

We use castor oil packs to remedy minor abdominal cramping, which is a folk treatment that works just as well now as it did a hundred years ago. Making one is simple: Cut an old flannel sheet into a square large enough to cover your trunk, up to the upper abdomen. Next, saturate the sheet with castor oil and warm it up. Place it across your trunk and leave in place until it cools, then place in a plastic bag and store in the fridge. You can use it a couple of times, but be sure to wear old clothes because the oil stains everything.

If adverse symptoms persist more than a few hours, contact your doctor immediately.

## Dry-Brushing Detox

Dry brushing—using a dry brush to stimulate your skin—opens pores, allows your body to breathe and enhances healthy organ function. In addition, brushing helps reduce the appearance of cellulite, fighting the dreaded fatty flesh problem. It tightens skin, aids digestion, reduces cellulite, stimulates circulation, increases cell renewal, cleanses the lymphatic system, removes dead skin layers, strengthens the immune system and stimulates the glands. All in all, this simple technique benefits the body both inside and out!

Use a natural vegetable-bristle brush; avoid synthetic materials, as they can irritate the skin. The brush should be kept dry and not used for bathing.

Dry brush right before you shower. It should take five or so minutes. Begin by brushing from your feet (bottom and over the top) toward the center of your body. Use sweeping, continuous short strokes. Then brush from your hands toward your chest, again using short sweep strokes. Brush in circular movements for an extra minute on problem areas such as your thighs (to help minimize cellulite), and then continue with other areas that need help.

A slight flushing of your skin is okay, but if it is red, you may be applying the brush too hard.

## DETOX Q&A

I asked Dr. Gloria Gilbére a few questions about cleansing, toxins and supplements for various skin problems. Here is what she had to say:

**BBG:** *Why should we cleanse?*

**GG:** For the same reason we should have our teeth cleaned by a professional: because brushing our teeth does not remove debris and plaque that accumulates over time and then causes decay and periodontal diseases. Cleansing the body removes accumulation of toxic matter that the body cannot do on its own on a regular basis, even though we drink plenty of water or have daily bowel eliminations.

**BBG:** *Why are we toxic?*

**GG:** Because our modern Western diets do not provide sufficient fiber to Roto-Rooter our intestinal system of accumulated debris that becomes health-depleting. In addition, modern diets contain additives, preservatives, flavor enhancers, coloring, and so on—all substances that are not natural to the body and inhibit its ability to neutralize or eliminate them.

**BBG:** *Should everyone cleanse?*

**GG:** Yes, even children—by making sure they drink plenty of clean water, eat fiber and eliminate daily.

**BBG:** *What is the best anti-aging method we can use?*

**GG:** Making sure our intestinal health is always at optimum, because science has validated that most of our immune system is based within our intestines. If anti-aging doesn't start from the inside out, any other protocols are strictly Band-Aids, and eventually they don't cover the effects of aging from the inside out.

**BBG:** *Why is it important to body brush?*

**GG:** It's important because the skin is the largest organ of elimination and absorption. Therefore, if we don't stimulate the pores to unclog trapped toxins, we cannot fully detoxify. Furthermore, skin brushing stimulates the lymphatic system to facilitate the elimination of toxic accumulation.

**BBG:** *Are there any concerns?*

**GG:** No, not with skin-brushing, unless someone brushes too deeply. Then it can cause skin irritation.

**BBG:** *Should we do it every day?*

**GG:** Yes, especially those with inflammatory conditions.

**BBG:** *Does it improve skin tone?*

**GG:** Absolutely! The analogy can be made that a beautiful piece of silver loses its luster when it becomes tarnished. Once polished, it again regains vitality. The skin is no different. It may not even have blemishes, but it loses its luster when toxic accumulation is not reduced.

**BBG:** *What about people with dry skin? Are there any herbs or foods that can help put the luster back in their skin?*

**GG:** The supplements I find that are best for the skin are vitamin C, CoQ10 [Coenzyme Q10] and plenty of pure water. The omega-3, -6 and -9 oils are also very important, as long as they are from a pure source.[21]

If you're not yet convinced that cleansing and detoxifying your insides promotes radiant health on the outside, consider this: Supermodel Kim Alexis is a devoted "detox-er." It seems as if she is always on some type of cleanse; she even has an infrared sauna in her home that she uses in the cooler months to aid in detoxification. Kim has regular colonics and loves to body brush in combination with a fitness routine and healthy eating. Now, I'm not saying that we'll all look like Kim Alexis after a good long cleanse . . . but if someone whose career is built on outer beauty focuses first on purifying her insides, that ought to be a good indication that it's important!

## EXERCISE TO DOWNSIZE

Remember the old commercial for a popular deodorant with the tagline "Never let them see you sweat"? Well, apparently many Americans have taken that commercial way too seriously. And "as a result, toxins and metabolic waste become trapped in the body instead of being released through sweat," says Dr. Gilbére.[22]

Improved physical health and fitness enhances inner and outer beauty, hands down. It is one of the key ingredients for anti-aging, and more importantly, your overall health. It also reduces stress, which we've already seen can greatly contribute to a toxic body.

There are so many options for exercising these days. You can go simple: Just head out for a healthy-cardio walk, jump rope or run. Lifting weights is also a great thing to do a few times a week to build muscle mass. You can join a gym or pop in one of hundreds of aerobic or weight-training DVDs. Find what works for you, but find something!

Here are a few more ideas to get you started.

### T-Tapp™

I'd like to plug a workout called T-Tapp, which is a comprehensive program created by fitness guru Teresa Tapp. She is an incredible woman with a real passion for helping people to be their best. Using T-Tapp, you reset your metabolism to burn at a faster rate, even if you occasionally cheat on your new lifestyle changes.

T-Tapp is an all-in-one workout that provides strength, body sculpting and cardiac conditioning. Its sequence of non-impact aerobic movements increases muscle strength and flexibility, improves bone density without weights, helps the body balance blood sugar and improves mental clarity. T-Tapp is a progressive workout designed to optimize neurokinetic (mind-to-muscle connection) and lymphatic function, which means that it works at a cellular level to help your body help itself by eliminating toxicity through the lymph system.

Teresa spent more than 18 years in the modeling industry as a new face developer. Part of her job was to help models get fit fast. She was able to utilize her T-Tapp workout for the models to use even when they were traveling because it can be done in as little as four square feet of space. The other really cool thing is that less is more; only one set of eight reps is needed for each exercise, and you don't have to do it every day to achieve results.

You can read more about T-Tapp in Teresa's book *Fit and Fabulous in 15 Minutes* or by visiting www.t-tapp.com.

## Yamuna Body Rolling™

Yamuna Body Rolling is a revolutionary approach to health and fitness using balls designed exclusively for this practice. YBR consists of a series of routines that use 6- to 10-inch balls to work specific muscles in detail, to create suppleness in tight areas and optimize range of motion.

Yamuna Body Rolling works like a hands-on practitioner, except instead of hands, balls are used to stretch muscles, dislodge tension and discomfort, increase blood flow and promote healing. Lying over the ball, you literally roll your body out, almost like dough, stretching and elongating your muscles. The YBR routines follow specific sequences that match the body's own logic and order; starting where each muscle begins, at its origin, you roll toward where it attaches, to the point called its "insertion."

I also appreciate that the balls are manufactured without chemical phthalates, which are commonly used in plastics and have been shown to have harmful health effects over time. To find out more about YBR, visit www.yamunabodyrolling.com.

## Rebounding

Looking back at my childhood, I realize that I used to do many beneficial exercises and never knew it, such as jumping on a trampoline outside in the fresh air. Who knew that the benefits far exceeded the fun? Today we call trampoline exercise "rebounding."

I had the chance to speak with Al Carter, who was a gymnastic trampoline professional during the 1970s. He is the pioneer of Rebound exercise and the founder of ReboundAIR, Inc. According to Al, "With each gentle bounce on the rebounder, approximately 60 trillion body cells are pitted against the Earth's gravitational pull. This interaction strengthens every cell in the body while saving strain on its muscles and joints."[23]

Here are just a few benefits of rebounding: (1) it increases the capacity for respiration; (2) it stimulates metabolism; (3) it circulates more oxygen to the tissues; (4) it helps normalize blood pressure; (5) it delays incidences of cardiovascular disease; (6) it aids lymphatic circulation, as well as blood flow in the circulatory system; and (7) it slows the aging process. That's something to jump for joy about! For more information, visit www.healthbounce.com.

## Pilates

Pilates is also a wonderful form of exercise that focuses on strengthening your core. Jackie Marushka, a publicist for artists such as Michael W. Smith, Third Day, Jars of Clay and Casting Crowns (to name a few), has a demanding job with a ton of responsibility. She knows, however, that her first responsibility is to herself. I met Jackie a couple of years ago backstage at the Dove Awards. I thought, *What a beautiful woman! She's healthy and glowing with such a vibrant personality.* I asked, "What is your secret to looking and feeling fabulous?"

Jackie pointed first to her faith in Christ, and then added, "As a publicist of 16 years, I've maintained a non-stop schedule filled with media visits, meetings and award shows. Being this busy requires a conscious effort to keep a balanced life. I have a spiritual mentor, I have learned how to eat well on the go, and I exercise. In an effort to add variety to my routine of running and weights, I turned to Pilates, and it's changed my life.

"As my core developed, my posture improved, my strength increased and the migraines and consistent neck tension I'd learned to live with ceased. . . . I wanted to share this with everyone who had ever struggled with stress, tension and neck and back problems. Sylvia, my incredible instructor, suggested I become certified to teach, so that while I was talking about the wonders of Pilates, I'd literally be able to walk someone through the process. I took the leap and got certified to teach."

If you suffer from some of the same stress-induced symptoms that Jackie was dealing with, Pilates may be the answer for you, too. For more information, visit www.powerpilates.com.

## LIFESTYLE CHANGE

Holly Wagner, founder of GodChicks ministry and author of *Warrior Chicks* and *Daily Steps for GodChicks*, made a complete lifestyle change after surviving breast cancer. She educated herself, seeking out resources to create a healthier lifestyle (her favorites include those by Jordan Rubin and Dr. Don Colbert). Holly decided to eat organically; she says, "I don't need pesticides in my body, and heavy metals were detected when I was tested." She now eats a lot of raw veggies and fruits and takes supplements.

Holly faithfully follows an exercise routine five to six days a week. "It is my responsibility to care for the one and only body God has trusted me with. I don't have the right to be careless of it. So to the best of my ability, I am going to eat the way I am supposed to and exercise. I am a capable woman. This has nothing to do with looking like a model; it's about longevity . . . about finishing your course."[24]

I couldn't have said it better myself. Holly is so right: We must not take our bodies for granted. I hope some of the suggestions I've offered in this chapter will help you begin to care for *your* one and only body from the inside out. I know I've given you a lot of information, but try not to be overwhelmed; changing even one of these aspects of your lifestyle will make a difference. Take it slow and add other anti-aging, positive, healthy changes into your life as you move forward, knowing that you are honoring God when you care for His gift of your body!

# Three

# Beauty 101: Skincare

As we flip through magazines, most of us see beautiful women with flawless skin and wonder, *How can I look like that?* Well, we all could if we had an army on our side: Commander Stylist laying out a strategy for perfection, Captain Makeup Artist brandishing his weapons of mass concealing, and Special Agent Airbrush covertly eliminating all enemy lines (not to mention a personal chef, massage therapist and trainer standing by). Any of us could grace the pages of a magazine with these warriors at our command.

Instead, most of us face the mirror alone, hoping that the products we just bought will "age defy" as promised. We know the basics—skin should be cleansed and moisturized daily—but every commercial we see, every magazine we read, every film or TV star promotes "the best" skincare products. How can *everyone's* products be *the best*? To compound the confusion, we also hear about "simple" skincare from women behind cosmetic counters and on infomercials and other media . . . and we would like a simple solution in our busy lives. But what, exactly, is "simple"? Inquiring minds want to know. Perhaps then we could face the mirror with confidence instead of fear.

If you're like so many other women, you know that skincare is important but you're not sure how to sort out fact from fad. Follow the skin-friendly guidelines in this chapter, and your body's largest organ will thank you!

## FACIAL CARE

The first step to creating your best skincare routine is to determine your skin's type and condition—are you sensitive, dry, oily, combination or acne-prone? The most effective way to determine your skin type is to visit a dermatologist or esthetician who can look at your skin under magnification, but if you don't have the means to see a professional, do it yourself with this simple test:

- Wash your face with tepid water.
- Wait one hour. Is your face feeling dry or slick?
- Use a lens or blotting tissue to press around your face (forehead, nose, cheeks and chin). If the tissue comes away dry and your pores appear small, then your skin does not produce very much sebum (oil); this means that your skin type is *dry*. If the tissue comes away oily and your pores appear larger, your skin produces more sebum; this means that your skin type is *oily*. If your face is oily only in the T-zone (forehead, nose and chin) and dry or normal everywhere else, you likely have *combination* skin. If you have medium-sized pores with smooth skin tone, your skin type is considered *normal*.

In addition to having skin that is normal, dry, oily or a combination, you may also have a skin condition that can influence the type of skincare products you choose. Let's take a quick look at these:

- *Sensitive skin* reddens from heat or irritation and may show allergic reactions to the sun or harsh products. The redness comes from dilated capillaries under the skin, often around the nose and cheeks, and it usually subsides after a short time.

- *Mature or aging skin* results from the passage of time and from hormonal changes.

- *Rosacea* is a chronic skin condition that begins with redness and flushing on the nose, cheeks and forehead, and may progress to papules or broken blood vessels, often during menopause.

Rosacea is aggravated by caffeine, spicy food, alcohol and extreme temperatures, and the redness usually does not subside completely unless medically treated.

- *Eczema* is a painful inflammatory skin condition that includes redness, itching, swelling, and dry or moist lesions. (Consult a dermatologist for an accurate rosacea or eczema diagnosis.)

- *Sensitized skin* is inflamed, itchy or tender due to pollutants, allergens and other irritants in the environment.

Your skin type and any skin conditions determine the kind of products you use for your daily skincare regimen.

## Cleanse

### Choose Your Cleanser

Don't spend a lot of money on a cleanser; you can use most any natural product, as long as it is right for your skin type. (Be sure to check out chapter 6 for a list of ingredients to avoid in skincare products.) For an alternative to cleanser, use the Wonder Cloth or Jane Iredale's Magic Mitt, both of which are made of microfibers and work with just water.

When choosing a cleanser for your skin type and condition, keep the following in mind:

- *Oily skin*: Use a sulfite-free gel cleanser—look for tea tree and/or rosemary as ingredients.

- *Dry skin*: Use a cream cleanser—look for rose and/or aloe as ingredients.

- *Mature skin*: Use a cream cleanser—look for rose and/or chamomile as ingredients.

- *Sensitive, sensitized or rosacea skin*: Use a cream cleanser—look for aloe, rose and/or chamomile as ingredients.

- *Normal skin*: Use a sulfite-free gel cleanser—look for lavender and/or rosemary as ingredients.

## Wash Your Face

Don't be a splasher. Most women wash their face for only 20 seconds, once a day. Twenty seconds can't possibly remove all the dirt, pollutants, makeup and oil from your complexion (and if you don't remove all of the junk, your pores may become permanently enlarged and may not shrink back!). Apply your cleanser to your face with your fingers as directed and then, using a sponge or soft washcloth, gently massage your skin to remove the cleanser. (You can also try the new brush by Clarisonic, though it's a bit pricey, or a facial brush for a couple of dollars.) In the evening, wash twice, first to remove makeup and then to banish the remaining funk. In the morning, assuming you have cleansed and moisturized the night before, you may wash only once.

**BBG TIP**

Chlorinated water can contribute to dry skin, so consider installing a shower filter. You will see and feel the difference.

## Exfoliate

Your skin needs regular exfoliation to slough off dead skin cells on the top layers of skin, making room for newer cells while not damaging new cell growth. Don't exfoliate more often than once a week. Dr. Ben Johnson, creator of Cosmedix and CEO of Osmosis Skincare, says that "chronic exfoliation can irritate, inflame, and swell the epidermis, which results in the false impression that the skin is getting younger and/or healthier. Furthermore, adding inflammation and damaging the epidermis makes the skin even less efficient and more starved for nutrients, which ultimately accelerates the aging process."[1] With that warning in mind, go easy on peels and other methods of intense exfoliation. Yes, they may have a temporary appeal, but later results may not be so pretty. If you do choose to exfoliate more often, be sure to wear extra sun protection afterward.

## Masks

Facial masks can exfoliate while also drawing out impurities and helping with other crucial needs of your skin. In addition, there is often immediate improvement in the feel and texture of your skin. Apply the product to your skin and let it dry at room temperature for several minutes (usually no more than 10 to 20). You will feel your skin tighten. Rinse off the mask, pat dry and apply moisturizer.

Some skincare lines, such as Eminence, offer masks for everyday use. Most, however, are best used only once or twice weekly to avoid irritation. You can also make your own mask. Any acidic ingredient will exfoliate and tone, while oils will nourish and hydrate. For instance, egg whites tighten skin, giving a temporary lift, while a mask of avocado nourishes and delivers intense moisture. (See chapter 7 for do-it-yourself mask recipes.)

### Facial Scrubs

I often hear skincare instructors advise that when you use a scrub, match the size of the granules to your pores. This is something you can determine on your next product hunt. I'm partial to scrubs containing jojoba beads, almond meal or oatmeal. Beware of apricot seeds and walnut shells, as they can be too harsh for delicate skin.

## Tone

Once your face is clean, you need to reset the pH balance of your skin. The pH is the degree of acidity or alkalinity of your skin or body; too low or too high a pH can cause inflammation or irritation. Your skin's pH should be between 4.5 and 6.2, and some products now carry the pH number on the packaging. Cleansers can make skin too alkaline, so get the pH balance back by using a toner designed for your skin type, or try a homemade toner from chapter 7, "The Pampered Pantry."

I don't think you need to spend a lot of money on toner; I use a simple rose spray from the health-food store. Just make sure the toner you choose is alcohol-free.

## Moisturize

Once your skin is cleansed and toned, it's time to add moisture back in. Be careful not to over-moisturize; many women apply too much moisturizer, which can clog pores and have negative rather than positive results. Use a pea-size amount of moisturizer for your face, a little extra for your neck and décolleté, and the size of a rice grain for your eyes (use a bit more if you have chronically dry skin). Apply in an up-and-out movement starting at the center of your face and neck.

You need a night moisturizer in addition to your daily moisturizer. This is usually a heavier crème and can include additional treatment ingredients. Applying at night allows the skin to absorb the crème over a longer period of time as you sleep.

### Eye Crèmes

Eye crèmes are highly concentrated and specially formulated to be multi-taskers, addressing fine lines, wrinkles, dark circles and puffiness. A good eye crème should be part of any anti-aging protocol, applied before you put on your all-over moisturizer.

Use your ring finger when applying eye crème (dot around the eye, following the eye muscle), as it is the weakest finger and won't apply as much pressure as others. This is a delicate area that should not be dragged or pulled; try "dotting" your eye crème instead of rubbing, to minimize pulling on the skin.

### Serums

A serum contains highly concentrated ingredients formulated into molecules much smaller than those in the average moisturizer, so it is absorbed more quickly and deeply. Similar to a moisturizer in design and purpose, a serum is a liquid meant to treat skin ailments such as dehydration, redness and fine lines. Think of it as a multi-vitamin for your skin, nourishing and protecting delicate cells from free radicals.

Depending on the serum's content, it may:

- firm and lift skin
- promote collagen production (reducing signs of aging)
- reduce the appearance of dark circles and puffiness in the eye area
- boost the skin's natural protection against environmental toxins
- stimulate circulation

Apply a drop of serum to your fingertips and massage gently into your freshly cleaned skin, morning and night, and then follow with moisturizer. You don't need to use more than a drop or two to cover your entire face and neck.

## LOOKING YOUNGER

All women want to look younger, but many don't start taking care of their skin early enough in life. I believe women should begin using mild anti-aging products as early as their late 20s, to keep their skin in better condition longer. The older your skin becomes, the more you need to include anti-aging ingredients in your skincare products.

### Anti-aging Ingredients

The anti-aging industry is growing so fast that it's hard to keep up with all the potentially useful products. Here are a few hints to help you navigate this growing market. As you shop, look for these natural ingredients in eye and face crèmes:

- *Hyaluronic acid* (or *sodium hyaluronate*): Keeps skin hydrated and looking full by drawing moisture from the air.

- *Antioxidants*: These include vitamin C, alpha-lipoic acid, green tea, milk thistle and coenzyme Q10, to name a few (a powerful antioxidant, COQ10 fights free radicals, thereby reducing wrinkles, discoloration and other texture changes).

- *Peptides*: Marine peptides and copper peptides are proteins that are easily absorbed by the skin, helping skin to appear more firm and stimulating growth of collagen and elastin.

- *Plankton extract*: Stimulates the production of collagen.

- *Argireline* (*hexapeptide 3*): Sometimes called the "Botox alternative," it relaxes wrinkles.

- *Argan oil:* This more recent addition to skincare products comes from the nut of the argan tree, grown in Morocco. "The oil, which is said to have restorative and age-defying effects, has become one of the latest miracle ingredients in the beauty industry. High in vitamin E and essential fatty acids, it is believed to help all sorts of skin conditions: dry skin, acne, psoriasis, eczema, wrinkles. Moroccans slather it on their skin, hair, nails and even their babies."[2]

- *Goji berry:* Rich in carotenoids and antioxidant vitamins C and E, goji berries fight the signs of aging and may help with dark under-eye circles.

GLOBAL BEAUTY TIP: KOREA

In Korea, women use the starchy, milky water from soaked white rice to wash their faces. The result is lighter-looking skin and a soft, dewy complexion.

## Facial Oils

French beauties of a certain age have sworn by these for years, and now many skincare lines are beginning to carry facial oils. I use them myself, and love the way they make my skin feel and look. Most contain carrier oils such as grapeseed, almond, primrose, avocado and others, while essential oils such as frankincense, sandalwood, lavender, neroli and other extracts help calm and nourish the skin. You can customize a personal blend for yourself with the recipe found in "The Pampered Pantry" (see chapter 7).

## Face Lighteners

Lighteners work on hyper-pigmentation and age spots and can lend an overall brightening to the face (though the effect is only temporary). When using lighteners, be diligent about using a good sunscreen (see below) because ingredients draw light to the skin. When shopping for a lightener, look for the following ingredients, as they are safer alternatives than hydroquinone, which is not good for your epidermis:

- Azelaic acid
- Kojic acid
- Lactic acid
- Arbutin

These are just a few of the many anti-aging ingredients currently available. You can find more listed in the Resources section, from companies with wonderful results-oriented skincare lines.

## Look Younger Tomorrow: 24 Tips

These natural approaches toward counteracting the effects of aging will work in less than 24 hours:

1. *Frownies.* These little tape devices work miracles without needles and have been around for a hundred years. Wear them at night or for at least four hours and you will see results. *Warning:* Your husband may think you look like a mummy.

2. *Make a mate latté.* Yerba mate tea tastes great and comes in many flavors. Heat water almost to boiling, steep for 10 minutes, strain, and then top it off with steamed, frothy milk (or use almond milk and a dash of cinnamon). Do not drink mate if you are taking an MAO inhibitor, as the combination may raise blood pressure.

3. *Positive attitude.* Various researches have shown that optimism increases good health. Start with positive self-talk: "I can handle this." Try to avoid criticizing yourself!

4. *Care for hands and feet.* Exfoliate (use the scrub recipe from chapter 7) and then, before bed, mix avocado oil and primrose oil in equal parts, apply a few drops to hands and feet, cover with gloves and socks, and go to sleep.

5. *Detox for a day* (see chapter 3).

6. *Dr. Gilbère's Seaweed Detox Bath.* This mineral bath increases blood and lymph flow to circulation-starved areas, breaks down

cellulite and moves waste out of your body. You can also use it as a body wrap.

7. *Whiten your teeth.* Try whitening strips while reading a book before you doze off.

8. *Sleep.* Get at least eight hours of sleep. Try to go to bed before 10 P.M. *Tip:* Listen to calming music for 45 minutes before bedtime. (I've heard of a study showing that music helped elderly folks sleep longer and feel less tired the next day. This may be because music decreases a key stress hormone in the body.)

9. *Sleep with a contour pillow,* the affordable alternative to pricey beauty pillows. The Anti-Wrinkle Pillow made by Eyetopia™ stretches the neck and reduces the pressure of face to pillow (which, in turn, reduces wrinkles!). Visit www.cynthiaboxrudmd.com for more info.

10. *De-stress with aromatherapy.* Try an inhalation sleep aid or make your own (see chapter 7).

11. *Use eye-hydrating goggles.* Saturate cotton pads with an herbal calming tonic such as argan or neem oil and place in these specially designed, hydrating goggles. Sleep in them or remove after 30 minutes. Visit www.dreamessentials.com to find out more.

12. *De-puff.* Cut back on white flour and sugar for 24 hours. Refined carbs cause your body to retain water, making your face "puffy."

13. *Pimple zapper.* Blend one packet of brewers yeast and a few drops of lemon juice and apply as a mask before bed. As the mixture hardens, it pushes away debris clogging your pores.

14. *Throw on another pillow.* Fifteen minutes before rising from bed in the morning, place an extra pillow under your head. This will help de-puff your eyes.

15. *Cut down on salt.* Salt makes you retain water. Avoid fast foods and switch to Spice Hunters, my favorite spices. My mom is now also a believer in these tasty salt-free spices.[3] (Those with

high blood pressure should only have 250 mg a day; the average person, 3,000 mg or less. If you are active and sweat a lot, you may need more.)

16. *Pray.* Thank God for everything before bed and before you get up. Be grateful!

17. *Be joyful.* A happy person looks younger because a smile sheds years.

18. *Get a pedicure and manicure, or DIY.* Soft hands and feet and clean nails are beautiful, with polish or without.

19. *Use a silk pillowcase.* Silk does not crease the way cotton does, and will not leave a mark on your face.

20. *Drink rooibos (red tea).* This South African tea has collagen-building copper, as well as vitamin C and other antioxidants.

21. *Enjoy a Sea Cal Bath by Spa Technologies.* Soak for 20 minutes in a blend of micronized coralaceous algae and marine plankton, rich in calcium and magnesium. These powerful minerals restore cellular balance by stimulating metabolism and eliminating excess water. Great for treatment of cellulite, water retention, PMS and bloating.

22. *Plump away your wrinkles.* Drink 8 to 10 glasses of water with lemon a day. Your skin will be more hydrated and the appearance of wrinkles less pronounced, while lemon helps with digestion.

23. *Avoid sugar.* It dries out your skin and promotes wrinkles.

24. *Choose an herbal coffee instead of a regular cup of joe.* In a coffee/tea press, make Teeccino Vanilla Nut caffeine-free herbal coffee, then mix with unsweetened vanilla almond milk, half a drop of Pure Inventions vanilla cocoa, and 1/2 tsp Xylitol—or add a little organic half-and-half (it's a vanilla-cocoa delight!).

When all else fails, live by what the wise Man said in Matthew 6:34: You've got enough problems for today, so don't worry about tomorrow. Or as we Italians like to say, "Fuggettabout it!"

## TREATING SKIN PROBLEMS

Special skin conditions require additional considerations beyond basic skincare. While you may need to consult a dermatologist for severe skin conditions, understanding some basic tips will help you reduce and manage these problems.

## Acne

While most often found in adolescent skin, many women continue to have problems with acne on into their 20s, 30s and beyond. Hormonal changes at various times of life can create acne conditions on the skin. It is important to consult a dermatologist for more severe cases, but even under the care of a doctor, follow these basic guidelines to reduce the severity and spread of acne.

### *Acne Don'ts*

1. *Don't over-cleanse.* Many people strip their skin by over cleansing their acned areas. When this happens, the body works harder and produces more sebum (oil), clogging pores and causing more acne. Clean your face at least twice, but no more than three times, a day.

2. *Don't touch.* Touching your face, especially with dirty hands and fingers, can aggravate an acne problem. No touching also means don't pick, squeeze or rub acne; doing so traumatizes the skin and slows the healing process, leading to more breakouts and even permanent scars and blemishes. Don't be conscious only of your hands . . . phones can also be dirty culprits against skin. Be sure to clean your cell phone, work phone and home phone often.

3. *Don't consume sugary foods or drinks.* Stay away from cakes, cookies, chocolates, candies, sodas and anything with refined sugar as a main ingredient. Sugar clogs pores and dries out and ages skin. Food allergies can also contribute to acne, as can certain medications (in particular, allergies to iodine-containing foods and the use of steroid inhalers).

4. *Don't use comedogenic products.* Skin with acne is battling an overproduction of sebum (oil), so don't exacerbate the problem by using oil-based moisturizers, facial crèmes or hair gels (hair often gets in the face, so don't use anything on your hair that you don't want on your skin!).

5. *Don't dry out acne in the sun.* Excessive sun exposure can tend to aggravate acne. UV rays destroy cells responsible for skin's immunology. I've seen some evidence that chronic sun exposure causes your pores to enlarge because it causes the sebaceous glands, oil-producing glands in your skin, to increase in size.

## Acne Dos

1. *Do increase your intake of fruits and vegetables.* Many natural foods are loaded with vitamins and minerals, which are some of the best acne fighters around. Green, leafy vegetables and orange- or yellow-colored fruits are rich in vitamin A, which inhibits overproduction of sebum. Oranges, strawberries, broccoli and lemon juice are some vitamin C-rich foods that fortify the body's defense system against acne-causing microbes, and aid faster healing of acne. Furthermore, vitamin C helps your body absorb vitamin E, which is essential for revitalizing and repairing damaged skin.

2. *Do drink lots of water.* Get the recommended 6-8 glasses of water a day. Drinking lots of water not only replenishes the body's water supply but also flushes out toxins that may cause acne.

3. *Do relax.* Stress, worry and pressure can disrupt your body's natural balance and lead to health problems such as acne. Getting a massage, going to the spa, taking a long bath, getting enough sleep or simply managing your time and schedule better are great acne treatments because they reduce acne-inducing stress.

4. *Do clean your gut.* Detoxing can improve acne tremendously. Be sure to consult with your doctor before starting any detoxification program.

5. *Do try natural remedies.* Azelaic acid has been shown to be comparable in results to benzoyl peroxide and other acne products, yet it is derived from wheat, barley and rye. Its antimicrobial action slows the growth of skin bacteria and appears to reduce skin redness, papules and pustules. Tea tree oil is also a great bacterial fighter, comparable to a 5-percent benzoyl peroxide, while essential oils such as neem and neroli are beneficial for oily skin.

## Rosacea

Some physicians see red skin or dilated capillaries and diagnose rosacea when it is actually sensitized skin that has been negatively impacted by environment. "Rosacea is a vascular disorder that includes flushing, small red bumps on or pustules on your nose, cheeks, forehead, and/or chin," says Denise Blair of the Dermal Institute. She goes on:

There's a female patterning and a male patterning of rosacea. So if it doesn't follow the patterning, then it probably is not rosacea; it's simply sensitivity. Skin can become sensitive genetically. Because of your Scottish-Irish or Celtic ancestry, you have fair skin, thinner skin, a higher histamine response, and a higher capillary response. Or your skin becomes sensitized due to environmental results, such as pollution, driving down the freeway with the backend of another car's exhaust in your face.[4]

GLOBAL BEAUTY TIP: SOUTH AFRICA

To soothe irritated and inflamed skin, women in South Africa steep a cup of rooibos, a tea leaf native to the area that contains zinc and alpha hydroxy acid. Allowing it to cool, they apply the liquid directly to the skin using a cotton ball. The tannins in the tea calm and relieve discomfort.

Some natural treatments for rosacea include niacinamide cream, chrysanthellum indicum (golden chamomile) cream, licorice (do not use if you have high blood pressure), rooibos (red teas), green tea, mallow, cucumber, ivy, sambuka and kokum butter (which has a high content of stearic-oleic-stearic-triglycerides, used to heal ulcerations and fissures on lips, hands and soles).[5] Red raspberry extract is a wonderful bioflavonoid that can strengthen capillary walls and minimize noticeable irritation. Oatmeal is also very soothing and can help reduce itching.

When dealing with sensitive, sensitized or rosacea skin, use the "less rule": less heat on your skin so you don't dilate the blood vessels, less manipulation, less product choices and less friction, which also causes vasodilation.[6]

Should you exfoliate with rosacea? "Yes," says Denise Blair. "One of the problems with rosacea is that the hydrophilic lipids barrier, commonly called the 'intercellular glue,' is damaged. There are breaks in that barrier's functioning. We want to keep that barrier functioning at optimal condition, and exfoliation helps to do that—gentle exfoliation, such as products containing rice bran."[7]

## BODY CARE

Your face is not the only place you have skin! But when most of us think about skincare, we think only of our face. We need to care also for the skin all over our bodies.

Be sure to use a pH-balanced body wash. So many bar soaps and cleansers can throw the body's pH out of whack. Our skin needs to maintain the correct pH to avoid inflammation or irritation. (See the Resources section for a helpful list of body washes with proper pH-balance.)

Just as you should exfoliate your face to slough off dead skin, you should exfoliate your body. Use products designed specifically for the body; particularly seek out natural scrubs such as salt- or sugar-based products. Again, avoid more abrasive ingredients (such as apricot seeds or walnut shells) to keep from damaging your skin.

Also, try the body-brushing technique described in the previous chapter. Brushing not only helps your whole body detox, but it's great for your skin as well.

## Fancy Feet

After walking several thousand steps a day, our feet endure a lot of travel time and need some TLC. Through the course of our lifetime, we will take enough steps to circle the globe several times over. That is a lot of pressure on a foot that has approximately 7,200 nerve endings, 26 bones, 20 muscles and hundreds of blood vessels—and we're just talking *one* foot here! With all that sole stomping, it's time to pamper our tootsies and show them some love.

Have you had a pedicure lately? This is a luxury that women deserve, and you can get one at a local cosmetology school for half the price of a spa or salon. Students are supervised by an instructor and are nearly finished with their esthetician program, so you can relax while you are being pampered, knowing that your feet are in good hands.

If your budget is tight or you don't like other people touching your feet, have no fear. With a basin near, paradise is on the way!

- Fill up a basin with warm water. Add a few drops of your favorite essential oil, such as lavender, and two tablespoons of baking soda.

- Use a foot file on your dry feet to remove dead skin and reveal baby-soft skin underneath (my favorite file is made by Microplane; visit http://us.microplane.com) or try the inexpensive and effective PedEgg.

- After you file, scrub your feet with a recipe from chapter 7, "The Pampered Pantry."

- Now place your feet in the basin and soak your soles for 10 minutes. Do not soak too long, as soaking can dry out skin.

- Pat dry, and then use a cuticle pusher to press back the skin around your toenails.

- Clip and file toenails squarely, in line with the ends of the toes, so that growth does not head into the surrounding soft tissue.

- Rub your feet with a few drops of sweet orange oil (mixed into a teaspoon of jojoba or grapeseed oil); it releases toxins in congested skin and helps in cell regeneration.

- Now that your feet are lubricated, massage the small toe joints between your index finger and thumb. Continue for one to two minutes per toe. Work toward the pad of your foot with your thumb in a caterpillar motion (thumb walking) and massage for a couple of minutes. (You can also try a foot massage ball—or even a tennis ball—to give your hand a rest!)

- With a wet Q-tip, dab around toenails to remove any excess oil. This will prepare the nail for polish.

- Polish your toes. Anise Cosmetics makes a nail polish formulated without formaldehyde, toluene and dibutyl phthalate. While nail polish is not natural, if you must wear it, use this brand or another formula such as Honeybees nail polish.

Now that your feet look and feel great, here are a few tips for making the feeling last.

- Sweaty soles? Use Summer Soles®, insoles designed to absorb sweat. All you do is peel and stick the product onto your shoe. Visit www.summersoles.com to find out more.

- Tired toes? Try YogaToes® Toe Stretchers. They stretch and separate toes while you relax. Visit www.yogapro.com for more information.

- Strengthen your toes and feet with Yamuna Foot Wakers®. These funky, spikey half-moons are designed to increase circulation, strength and flexibility in your feet. Order at www.yamunabodyrolling.com.

- Teresa Tapp has a foot fitness DVD that can be taken anywhere—and you don't need any equipment! Find it at www.t-tapp.com.

Our feet endure stress, pressure and pain from tight shoes, bad walking habits and standing in one place for long periods of time. We must remember to give our soles a break! Change shoes after wearing for several hours, keep feet hydrated, seek out a podiatrist for checkups, and have a pedicure (or do one at home) at least once a month.

God gave us these feet to walk with Him, and to take care of ourselves and the ones we love. Sit down, relax, put your feet up and thank God for your soles!

## Healthy Hands

Now that we've pampered our feet, let's not forget about the hands. As you may already know, hands tend to show age, develop brown spots, dry out and get sun damaged earlier and more easily than other parts of the body. At the same time, our hands are very noticeable parts of us, so give them a little care and tenderness to keep them at their best. Here are a few tips:

- If you suffer from dry hands, use gloves while washing dishes, cleaning and especially while working in the garden.

- Avoid harsh cleansers and antibacterial washes. Recent studies have shown antibacterial products don't work well and can leave your hands very dry.

- For a quick fix, slather on Un-Petroleum Jelly made by Avalon Organics, then put on cotton gloves for at least two hours, or overnight. (If you want to treat hands while cleaning house, add a pair of snug-fitting latex gloves over the cotton ones.)

- You can get a microdermabrasion treatment at the spa and pay $75, or you can choose the healthier (and cheaper!) way at home. Soak your hands in an herbal hand bath treatment (see chapter 7 for the recipe). Apply a natural-ingredient exfoliant to your hands, rinse, and then apply the mask you use on your face. Leave on for 20 minutes, rinse, and then apply a spot lightener (you can use your face lightener) and finish with a moisturizer.

- Take care of your cuticles by using a cuticle oil, either home-made (see chapter 7) or made with natural ingredients, such as Burt's Bees® Lemon Butter Cuticle Crème.

## SKIN'S WORST ENEMY

Ninety percent of skin damage and aging is caused by the sun's UV radiation, and 50 to 80 percent of the damage is done before age 18.[8] However, much of this damage is preventable. By wearing hats, protective gear and sunscreen, UV exposure is almost entirely controllable.

Denise Blair from the Dermal Institute says that we should wear sunscreen every day over the entire body, not just exposed skin. A shirt only gives a 2-percent SPF, and we are constantly exposed to ambient sunlight, such as through the window in the car or office. Ten minutes of ambient sunlight every day for a month is equivalent to five hours at the beach.[9]

When it comes to choosing a sunblock or sunscreen, there are many products on the market. What ingredients should you look for to ensure your sun protection is effective?

*Sunblock* usually contains zinc oxide or titanium dioxide, which are effective protection against both UVA and UVB rays that cause sunburn and can lead to skin cancer. Sunblocks are "full-spectrum" because they protect from all UV rays. Zinc and titanium are the only FDA-approved physical sunscreens, and they are both naturally occurring minerals.

*Sunscreen*, on the other hand, usually contains oxybenzone (or dioxyboenzone) to protect from UVB rays, and avobenzone to protect from UVA rays. Both are chemicals (which I prefer to stay away from). Avobenzone-containing products have decreasing efficacy after a few hours of sun exposure, but the addition of oxybenzone reduces the amount of degradation that occurs.

Sensitive skin does especially well with full-spectrum sunblocks titanium dioxide or zinc oxide (because chemical sunscreens can be skin irritants), but I recommend them for every skin type and condition. There are questions about potential harm from chemical suncreens over time, and I think it's better to stick with natural minerals approved by the FDA as effective. (Many women have begun to use mineral makeup because these products are generally SPF 18 or higher.) Whether you choose a sunblock or a sunscreen, shoot for SPF 15 or higher. Today, most moisturizers are SPF 8 or higher (especially tinted moisturizers), and you can combine yours with a low-SPF sunblock to exceed SPF 15. (See the Resources for the top-10 sunscreens from the EWG.)

Purchase and regularly wear a *fun*ctional, fashionable hat with a UPF of 50+ (equal to an SPF of 30) and fabulous sunglasses with UV400. With this combined protection, you can feel confident out in the sun, whether you're gardening, beachcombing or simply taking a walk. Some of these products are available online (see the Resources section).

## WHEN BEAUTY EXPIRES

Just about every consumable has an expiration date, right? Why is it, then, that we rarely consider the expiration of cosmetics and toiletries, considering we put them in our hair and on our skin? According to the FDA, cosmetics aren't required by law to have expiration dates (you can't just look at the label to know when a product should be retired), but that doesn't mean they will last forever. Everything has a shelf life, especially natural products!

**BBG TIP**

Nifty little gadgets called Timestrips® can be attached to your cosmetics to tell you when it's time to toss. (No, they won't help you stay on time while putting on your makeup, but wouldn't that be cool?) Visit www.timestrip.com for more info.

So how do we pay attention to the "use by" dates of our skincare products and cosmetics? Thankfully, some companies are now labeling their products with dates, but be aware that these are simply a guide; a product's safety may expire long before the label's date if the product has not been properly stored. For instance, cosmetics exposed to high temperatures or sunlight—or opened by consumers prior to purchase—

may substantially deteriorate before the expiration date. Once you open your new product, airborne bacteria swarm in. You add to that bacteria if you touch the product with unclean hands or applicators. Even if you use products with bacteria-fighting preservatives (avoid them unless they are plant-based!), aging cosmetics lose the battle with bacteria over time. (Speaking of bacteria . . . think about testers located at department store cosmetic counters! People constantly stick their hands in the makeup and try it on without asking for help. If you decide to try a product tester, make sure pencils are sharpened and fresh tools are used when makeup is applied.)

The question then is, *How long can we keep our little hopes in the bottle, and can we extend their shelf life to protect ourselves from infections such as pink eye and skin breakouts?* Below are some guidelines for expiration dates and tips for shelf-life extension:

## Color Makeup

Mineral makeup in powder form has no expiration. However, unwashed brushes may bring bacteria into the mix, so dispose of opened containers after two years, at most.

Liquid foundation lasts three to six months. Crème foundation can last four to six months. Foundation in a pump dispenser will last a little longer, because it is less exposed to air than foundation in a jar. If it has a higher percentage of pigment, such as in liquid or crème mineral makeup, it will last about 12 months. *Here's a tip*: Using the front of your hand as a palette, squirt a small amount of product onto your hand and apply to your face with a disposable applicator.

Concealer has a shelf life of six to eight months. Powders, including eye shadows and blush, last 12 to 24 months. Mascara lasts for three months. *Hint:* Never pump your mascara; air just pushes back into the tube, drying it out and inviting bacteria. Clean your wand with tissue every couple of days to prevent clumping. Lip gloss and lipstick have a shelf life of one year. Eye and lip pencils will stay fresh for 12 to 18 months with continued sharpening; you will know it has gone bad when it crumbles.

## Skincare Products and Body Washes

Facial cleansers and moisturizers can keep for about six months, unless they contain acids such as glycolic acid, salicylic acid and beta hydroxyl acid. Then they have a longer shelf life. Try putting eye crème in the fridge; it feels great on tired eyes and may slightly improve shelf life (or check out a "cosmetic cooler" to keep your products free of heat-loving bacteria).

Facial toner should be thrown away after 12 months, but if it contains vitamin C, the nutrients may lose potency before that time. Natural body washes last for six months.

## Applicators

Brushes should be washed regularly, as often as once a week, with mild soap and warm water. You can use alcohol; it's a little harsh, but it works in emergencies. You may also use a spray brush cleaner. Makeup sponges need to be cleaned after every use. Toss within a month or when sponges show wear and tear.[10]

As the old saying goes, "When in doubt, throw it out" . . . especially if there's no date on the label!

## SIMPLE SKINCARE

For *simple* skincare, you gotta K.I.S.S.—Keep It Super Simple. Follow these basic steps: cleanser, toner, serum, moisturizer, sun protection. Once a week, apply your mask and/or exfoliant and you are good to go.

And remember this: Aging is not a disease; it is a privilege. As we grow older, we can spread wisdom and joy to those around us. We can mentor the young and help the old. We can watch our kids grow. The most beautiful thing we can do is share our past mistakes and future hopes with women around us to show them God's love. True beauty is simple and simply has no limits!

# Four

## Face Forward:

### Steps to a Flawless Face

n some circles, makeup can be a bit controversial. Some say that makeup is just a façade—that cosmetics are superficial. Others may even say that wearing makeup is a sin. Still others are more pragmatic: A pastor once said from the pulpit, regarding his view on makeup, "Well, if the barnyard door needs a painting, then give it a coat or two." Not too flattering, but he made his point.

No matter what the opinion on makeup, I have seen it change women dramatically. Not too long ago I gave a makeover to a young missionary woman at a conference who had never had her makeup done. Growing up without a mom had left her clueless about a basic skin-cleansing routine, much less how to apply makeup. What a sweet spirit she had, and getting to know her was a delight as I taught her a few simple techniques. When I was done, she looked in the mirror and began to cry. I thought, *Oh, no . . . what did I do?!* But then she turned to me with tears in her eyes and said, "Thank you." Looking back in the mirror, she exclaimed with surprise in her voice, "I look beautiful."

"You *are* beautiful," I confirmed. Her quiet wonder proved once again that a little change on the outside can drastically change how we feel on the inside.

Another woman at that conference was in the middle of a divorce and was readying herself to reenter the workforce. She needed a change to boost her confidence. After our makeup session, she looked in the mirror and remarked with tears in her eyes, "Now I feel like I can do this." She hadn't felt good about herself in years.

I know that makeup is not *the* answer and that ultimately we must ground our confidence in God. However, for some women, simple outer changes can be a catalyst for greater inner shifts, just as inward transformation is often revealed by outward improvement.

Before you get started, make sure you keep the following tools handy for the smoothest makeup application possible:

- Latex-free sponge
- Flock sponge
- Powder brush (large brush for powder)
- Blush brush (angled or rounded to apply blush)
- Concealer brush
- Fine detail brush (for eyeliner)
- Lip brush
- Powder puff (velour)
- Small fan brush (from art supply store)
- Crease brush (for eye shadow)
- Flat eye shadow brush
- Eyelash curler
- Tweezers
- Q-tips
- Baby wipes

## LAYING THE FOUNDATION

Take care what you use and how you apply it. Paying attention to your products and learning some simple application tips can make all the difference in creating the right look for you. (Remember, looking like a member of the rock group KISS is not what we're going for!)

Makeup is an extension of skincare. Once you've established a healthy skincare routine, the next step is to find the right makeup . . . and your foundation sets the "foundation" for the rest, like preparing a canvas for the artist's masterpiece. With that in mind, choose products that are free from preservatives and carcinogenic ingredients (see chapter 6 for a list of the ingredients to avoid). Your skin needs to breathe, and if you put a bunch of unhealthy goop on your face, it will suffocate!

> Before you apply foundation—powder or liquid—apply a primer, which will help minimize pore size. Some brands also help reduce shine. Wait one to two minutes, and then apply your foundation (if you put the foundation on too soon, your skin will appear uneven in color).
>
> **BBG TIP**

Without building a smooth and proportioned foundation underneath a house, the outcome would be a disaster, right? The same goes for the structure of your face. Begin with the right foundation to avoid a makeup disaster. Let me give you a brief overview of your options:

- *Stick* foundation also acts as a concealer and is best for normal-to-dry skin, giving women more coverage.
- *Liquid* foundation is the most common and fits most skin types.
- *Crème* foundation is smooth and is formulated for dry-to-normal complexions.
- *Mousse* foundation is a crème that has a whipped consistency. Great for mature skin because it is less noticeable in fine lines.
- *Tinted moisturizer* is moisturizer with pigment. It's the sheerest of all foundations. It evens out skin tone while providing minimal coverage.
- *Crème-to-powder* foundation has a creamy texture that dries to a powder finish. It provides a matte finish on oily skin.
- *Powder compact* is a dual-finish powder foundation and can be used wet or dry. Great for young women because it's low in oils and doesn't clog pores.

- *Mineral powder* comes loose or pressed and now also in liquid form. It works much like a dual-finish powder foundation and is simple to apply. Pressed powder works best for oily skin, while more mature skin looks best with loose powder. (*Note:* Bismuth oxychloride, a common ingredient used to bulk up cosmetic powders, has a low toxicity, but it can occasionally cause allergic reaction and makes skin look shiny—it happens to make my skin itch.)

**BBG TIP**

When choosing a color, select one shade lighter than your skin in a loose powder. Pressed and liquid are usually right on color target. If your complexion is oily or you have darker skin, choose a liquid one shade lighter than your skin (oil turns foundation darker over time, as it oxidizes).

## Find Your Shade

Sometimes it seems as if finding the right shade of foundation is like finding that perfect shoe—do they really exist?! Yes. (And maybe the shoes do, too.) Before choosing your color, you need to know your skin tone. Are you warm or cool? Here is a quick test to determine your tone:

- Warm skin tone has greenish veins and burns easily—gold looks better on you.
- Cool skin tone has bluish veins—silver looks better on you.

When testing your shade choices, place three different swabs of color on your face between the cheek and jawline. The one that disappears into the skin is your color. Keep in mind that your color will not always be the same as it was in high school—your skin does change as you get older.

## Conceal

Some concealers, depending on the ingredients, accentuate lines rather than obscure them. Ingredients to look for are vitamin K, green tea extract and jojoba esters to help repair blood vessels and camouflage signs of fatigue. Dark circles may be genetic rather than a result of too little sleep or too much stress, but plenty of rest and a good concealer will go a long way.

My favorite concealer color is light peach to salmon (sometimes slightly golden), depending on skin tone. If the concealer is too dark, it can accentuate the problem; too light, and it produces a grayish cast.

I use the same motion applying concealer as when I put on eye crème: Dot under the eye following the eye muscle, ending under the outside corner of the eye (a little below the lash line). Sometimes I do the lid, too. This is a delicate area, so use a concealer brush to spread the concealer, then blend well. The fingers work too and can warm up the product, but be sure not to drag the skin.

## Create Contours

If you have specific issues with the appearance of your face, such as wanting to slim your nose or emphasize your cheekbones, you can use a technique called *contouring*—using color to create shading on various parts of your face. You can also even out skin tone using light and dark shades of foundation.

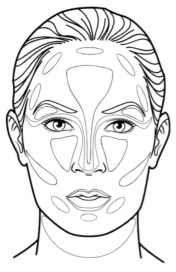

I learned my favorite method of contouring from my friend and fellow makeup artist Eve Pearl.[1] She suggests using three color foundations: one that matches skin tone, one that is two shades darker (for defining and contouring) and one that is two shades lighter (for highlighting).

Apply the lightest shade to the T-zone (forehead, nose, part of cheek and around lips). Now use the medium shade (the one that matches your skin) on the rest of your face.

The next step is a little tricky: Using a concealer brush or sponge for the darker shade, carefully shape hollows in your cheeks, over your jawline and under your chin (if you want to camouflage that area). Then, using a clean sponge, blend the darker shade with a patting motion.

Final step: Set the foundation with loose or pressed powder to seal in place. One of my favorite tools for this final job is a powder puff. Fold the puff like a taco, dip into your powder and then rub the puff's side to get rid of excess. Using a rolling motion, work the powder into skin.

## Blush

Add blush to cheeks, forehead and sides of nose for the finishing touch. I have found crème blush works best for dry or mature skin. Unlike powder, which sits on top of the face, crème blush melts into the skin and gives a dewy, more natural look. For both crème and powder, think rosy—apply on the apples of your cheeks and blend to revive your complexion.

# EYES: THE WINDOWS TO YOUR SOUL

Your eyes are often the first thing people notice about you, so apply eye makeup that will enhance, not overshadow, the windows to your soul.

## Primer

Prime eyelids first. This keeps the area matte so your other shadows last throughout the day. I use a lemony color over the entire eyelid—use concealer or powder if you're in a hurry. If you choose a crème lid primer, go over the eyelid with your powder puff afterward, lightly pressing into the skin.

## Eyeliner

### Powder

Start with a clean flat-edged or angled brush. Place a dab of water on the top of your hand, dip the tip of your brush into the powder and then into the water to make a crème, and then apply the coated brush to your lash line—from inner corner to outer corner—in a series of dashes. Seal the deal with a cotton swab along the top line to soften the effect.

### Liquid

Apply liquid eyeliner with your eyes open. Draw a short line at the beginning, middle and end of your lid and then connect the lines.

*Pencil*

Be sure your pencil is sharp. Use the same approach as with a liquid, but when you pencil the bottom eyelid, start from the outside corner and line halfway in; then use a Q-tip or a smudge tool to ever-so-lightly go over the hard line. This softens the line and also makes the end result more natural.

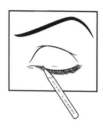 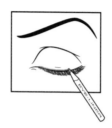 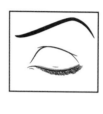

## Eye Shadow

Use a light shade to cover the entire eyelid area. With a darker shade, make a sideways V (>) pointing to the outside of your eyelid and opening toward the middle. Follow with the lighter shade on the inside corner of your eye and your brow bone. You may use a highlighter color, such as a creamy pearl or pearl pink, below the eyebrow to brighten your eye.

## Lovely Lashes

Aren't you glad you weren't born in 3000 B.C.? I read once that the ancient Egyptians applied kohl—soot blended with crocodile dung, warm donkey liver and honey—to their lashes with tiny sticks. Hmmmm . . . let me think about this: the smell, the pain, the goo? The price of beauty was steep. (The Egyptians also used crocodile dung as a contraceptive, which sounds pretty effective!)

The final touch in making up your eyes is mascara, which is no longer made, thankfully, of crocodile dung. Before applying mascara, use an eyelash curler to curl your lashes; this will make them stand out even more. (My favorite curler is made by Shu Uemera, but in a pinch I have used a pencil by wrapping lashes around the barrel and applying mascara at the same time.) After curling, use a lash conditioner, which helps to lengthen and condition.

Now you're ready for mascara. Start from the base of the lash and jiggle your way through to the tips, then do one complete sweep from the lash base. As for bottom lashes, I suggest using a tiny fan paintbrush (find one at an art supply store). Dip the fan brush in mascara and slightly sweep bottom lashes (or just leave them bare).

## EYEBROWS: FRAME TO FAME

There I was at a writer's conference, doing makeovers and shaping eyebrows in my hotel room. There were knocks on my door at all hours of the day and night, from women sneaking in to get their eyebrows done and makeup touched up. An amazing fiction writer (who shall remain nameless) told me that she needed a new headshot and had never waxed her eyebrows . . . ever. As I offered her a seat, I thought, *I love first-timers.* "Well, this will feel a little warm," I told her as I spread the melted wax across her brow. Then I added, "Have you ever had a baby?" and applied pressure to the strip of Pellon.

"Yes . . ." she admitted hesitantly.

"Good . . . then you know what pain is."

*Riiiiip* . . . I pulled out the unwanted hairs. She gasped and laughed, all at the same time, as I proudly showed off my kill. Caterpillar no more.

To some, this may sound like a horror story, but as the saying goes, "No pain, no gain." (True horror would be waiting in the salon for the esthetician and then thinking when you see her half-moon eyebrows, *Those*

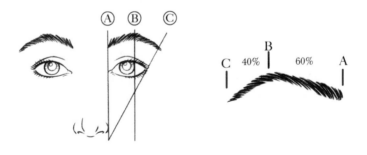

*commas belong in a sentence, not above your eyes!* Then she says, "I'm going to shape your brows just like mine." Run away!)

Seriously, beautiful eyebrows can take years off your face by allowing your eyes to be more of a focus. Most makeup artists agree that brows are one of your most important facial features. Marvin Westmore of Westmore Academy, Hollywood's premiere makeup artist and eyebrow expert, sees the eyes as the framework of the face. He has a great eyebrow technique that I managed to master over some time.[2]

Here we have the 60/40 Rule for the proper length and dimensions of your eyebrow: From point A to point B = 60 percent; from point B to point C = 40 percent.

Hold a brow pencil vertically alongside your nose; where the inside of the pencil meets the brow is where your eyebrow should begin. Mark the spot (A) with a white eyeliner pencil. The arch of your brow should be outside your iris; mark that spot (B) as well. Then mark the end of your eyebrow (C), which should be just past the outer corner of your eye. (If you need extra help, try using a brow stencil to help you get the right shape. Some brow stencils that work: Anastasia All About Brow Kit, Alexis Vogel eyebrow stencils, and Ardell Eyebrow Perfection Stencils. You're ready for the red carpet!)

Now that you have an idea of the shape you want, tweeze one hair at a time to fit the dimensions you have outlined. (No time to tweeze? Use a brow razor, which can be found at any beauty supply store.) The outer 40 percent of the brow should end in a slight upsweep. This upsweep opens the outer side of the eye and gives a more harmonious shape to the brow when viewed from the front.

> If you have unruly brows, apply castor oil with a Q-tip. This will smooth brows and has been known to stimulate hair growth, as does emu oil.

**BBG TIP**

If your brow hairs are long, trim rather than tweeze. Brush them upward and then cut with brow scissors to create a layering effect. This will lay brows flat so they don't stick out.

If you use an eyebrow pencil, be sure it is sharp. Use light, feathery strokes; don't draw a solid line. I prefer to use a powder shadow rather than a pencil, but tinted brow gel works well too (or use clear gel after applying pencil or shadow). For a bit more drama, highlight brows with gold mascara in place of brow gel, or mix a bit of gold eye shadow or powder with hair wax or pomade and then brush through the brows. Voilà!

I asked Marvin what color brows should be, in terms of darker or lighter than one's natural hair color. His response was, "Not darker or lighter. Taupe is my general preferred color, then blonde, then midnight brown [gray-brown]."[3] However, the late makeup artist Kevyn Aucoin suggested that brunettes and redheads should choose a shade lighter than their natural brow color and blondes should go for a slightly darker shade. Obviously, eyebrow shade is a matter of taste. Try several different shades and see what looks best to you.

## BEAUTIFUL LIPS

You've worked your way to the final touch on your facial work of art: your lips. Creating the right look for your lips is a crucial step; don't leave it to the last minute, using the rearview mirror to throw on your lipstick be-

### Secrets of a Celebrity Makeup Artist

Eve Pearl is a five-time Emmy Award winning celebrity makeup artist, and the author of *Plastic Surgery Without the Surgery: The Miracle of Makeup Techniques*. Here are a few of her tricks of the trade:

- Applying a hint of gold below the eyeliner toward the outer eye will make eyes pop.
- When you use your puff, dip a little extra loose powder and apply just below your blush; this too will create more definition.
- If you've applied too much blush, smooth it out by blending away the edges with a neutral or light powder at the edges.

fore jumping out of the car! Lip color can make or break your total look, so take care.

## A Mini History of Lipstick

Lipstick has been around for thousands of years, dating back to ancient Babylon, when semiprecious jewels were crushed and applied to the lips and occasionally around the eyes. (I guess that's where cosmetic companies came up with glitter eye shadows.) Egyptian Queen Cleopatra's lipstick

*Did you know....?*

❋ Carmine—also called crimson lake, cochineal, natural red 4, C.I 75470 and E120—is a bright red pigment obtained from the carminic acid produced by some scale insects.

was made from carmine beetles, which provided a deep pigment, added to a base of smashed ants. (I draw the line at the ants. This must have been the early version of *Fear Factor*.)

Queen Elizabeth I wore bold red lipstick on her pale face in the sixteenth century, and by the 1920s, many common women welcomed red lips as a symbol of their newfound power and voice. In the 1930s, the most popular shade was a deep oxblood hue, and some said kissing went out of fashion due to the high cost of lipstick. In the '50s, paler lips came and went, giving way to strawberry meringue—thanks to Max Factor—in the

- For a more natural look, outline your lips with a shade lighter than your lipstick.
- Create more dramatic eyes with false eyelashes.
- To tame the tricky under-eye area, use concealer in these tones:
  - ◆ On light/medium skin with bluish veins, use light peach/salmon
  - ◆ On medium/dark skin, use honey yellow/salmon/orange
  - ◆ On dark purplish circles, use yellow/light peach/salmon
  - ◆ On dark brown/reddish spots, use yellow/light peach

'60s. The natural look was popular in the mid-to-late '70s, but heavier makeup was all the rage in the 1980s, with red lips once again.[4]

Basically, women have been puckering up for centuries, no matter the cost.

## Lipstick Shades

Personally, I am not a big fan of dark lipstick, at least not on me. Nothing ages you like dark lips, especially if yours are already on the thin side. *Lighter emphasizes, darker minimizes.* If you are old enough to have adult children, stick to lighter colors on your lips. Here are some good color choices according to your shade of hair and skin:

- *Redheads*: peach, apricot, warm pink, sheer coral, honey-colored nude and raisin

- *Blondes*: pink, mocha pink, peachy pink, sandy pink, rose and golden raspberry

- *Brunettes*: rose, berry, plum, bronze, golden pink, browny pink, sheer coral, wine and shimmery mocha

- *Mocha skin*: beige, sheer gold, coffee, caramel, berry, plum, wine, pink, sheer raisin, coral and bronze

- *Dark skin*: warm camel, coffee, toast, deep bronze, true crimson, burnished plum. Also go for glosses in hues such as gold, golden chestnut and deep sheer berry

If you find red irresistible, follow these guidelines: Fair skin tones should wear blue-based pinks and reds, while medium skin tones look great with orangey shades. Dark skin tones can use any shade as long as it is bright enough to show up. Blue undertones will make your teeth look whiter, or you can use whitening strips, baking soda or the Rembrandt Whitening Pen to brighten your teeth.

When choosing a lipstick, look for natural ingredients. Some brands may contain lead, and the higher the lead count, the greater the risk to your health (see chapter 6 for other ingredients to avoid).

## Lip Preparation

Now that you have chosen a lip color and your teeth look great, you need smooth lips. Cracked lips can make you look older, so avoid them!

Before applying lipstick, gently exfoliate your lips with olive oil or lip balm on an old toothbrush. Or mix up your own exfoliant from brown sugar and almond oil, then massage into lips.

## Lip Application

### *Lip Liner*

You can do this a couple of ways, depending on the effect you want: (1) Fill in where you need it. If your top lip is fading and thinning, fill just outside the lip line with dashlike strokes. If you need more help on the bottom, do the same for the lower lip. If you need definition on the whole mouth, apply on top and bottom. Just remember to use dashlike stokes instead of drawing a solid line; this method will soften the results. (2) Jane Iredale uses a terra-cotta lip liner (from her product line) to make short strokes on the lip line and then fill in with feathery strokes at the corners, top and bottom. This leaves a small space to apply an opal-colored eye shadow on the cupid's bow and the middle of the lower lip, giving lips a plumper look. Top it off with gloss (Jane uses tourmaline).

*Did you know...?*

❄ The lipstick plant (also know as aeschynanthus) has red tubular buds and is native to Indonesia, New Guinea and the Philippines.

### *Lipstick*

After applying liner, fill in with lipstick, preferably using a lip brush to smooth the color on, and blend with liner.

#### Six Steps to Long-Lasting Lip Color

1. Apply a light layer of foundation to your lips.

2. Wait a few seconds, then pat lips with loose powder.

3. Outline lips with liner and fill in with feather-light strokes.

4. Blot with tissue.

5. Apply lip color with brush to the center first, working toward edges.

6. Blot with tissue (lightly—you don't want to smudge your masterpiece).

## BBG TO GO

Every woman needs a small makeup kit in her purse for touching up on the go. Here are my suggestions to include in your beauty-to-go bag:

1. Instead of carrying foundation, choose a concealer to cover up circles and blemishes and to touch up on the go.

2. Put color in your bag, such as a multipalette with lip, cheek and eye colors.

3. Lip liner: nude, spice or terra-cotta

4. Lip balm, such as the one from Burt's Bees, or make your own (see chapter 7)

5. Eyelash curler and mascara

6. Tweezers

7. Oil blotter tissue paper

When you only have a minute or two (or five), follow these basics to get yourself looking your best in a time crunch.

### The Two-Minute Face

1. Apply tinted moisturizer all over your face.

2. Curl eyelashes, then apply mascara.

3. Apply bronzer on eyes, cheeks and lips.

4. Dab on lip balm.

## The Five-Minute Face

1. For mineral powder foundation, use a kabuki brush to apply all over face. For liquid, use a sponge to apply over face.

2. Using a camouflage brush, spot conceal where needed, including on nasal folds, redness.

3. Apply blush on apples of your cheeks.

4. Line your lashes with pencil or slanted brush.

5. Curl eyelashes, then apply mascara.

6. Line lips with short dashes, and fill in lip color to dazzle.

*The best makeup of all is joy!*

I hope these product and application tips have given you confidence to create the right look for your face. Enhancing what God gave you on the outside can boost your confidence on the inside, but never forget that true confidence—just like true beauty—comes from knowing that God created you as a uniquely beautiful woman with much more than your face to offer the world.

# Five

# Haute, Healthy Hair

N ow your beautiful face needs a frame. But great hair is not just about products, tools and chemistry; those factors probably account for 90 percent of your hair and style, and the other 10 percent is creativity. (The good news is that you don't have to spend a fortune on styling products; you can even make some of them in your own kitchen. See chapter 7.) In this chapter, you'll learn how to care for your hair with the right products and tools, while smart tips from celebrity stylists will help you look your best.

The Bible says that the hairs on your head are numbered, describing how much God cares for you (see Luke 12:7). Hair, for most of us, is one of our most defining characteristics. We vary the color and length of our hair to describe ourselves to others. We use our satisfaction (or dissatisfaction) with it as a benchmark for our contentment with the rest of our appearance. (How many of us say that we're "having a bad *face* day"?)

Whether you're having a good or bad hair day, your hair is primarily made of keratin, the same protein that is the foundation of your nails, teeth and skin. Each strand of hair is about 97-percent protein and 3-percent moisture, a ratio that makes it essential to nurture your tresses. Caring for your hair includes cleansing, moisturizing and choosing a style that suits your face, personality and lifestyle. But where do you begin?

## START WITH YOUR HAIR TYPE

Hair care products can be confusing. Standing in the hair-care aisle at the store can be overwhelming—so many choices for so many different things!—but just because your friend or sister uses something, that doesn't mean that it's right for you. Start by knowing your hair type and any needs specific to your hair. These factors should determine the type of products you need. Whatever your type—dry, oily, normal, combination or fine—make sure you choose appropriate pH-balanced shampoos and conditioners.

**Coarse hair.** Choose shampoos with olive oil and/or wheat germ. Coarse hair gets fuzzy and wiry after cleansing, so look for serums or leave-in conditioners to seal and smooth.

**Curly hair.** Choose shampoos that maximize curls. Curly hair tends to be frizzy, so leave-in conditioners and shine enhancers or conditioning sprays help.

**Black hair.** This type of hair is usually dry and brittle, so use a hydrating shampoo with conditioners. Look for those with ingredients such as shea butter and jojoba oil.

**Chemically treated hair.** Choose shampoos with shea butter, olive oil, pro-vitamin B and/or green tea. Hydrate hair by using products with moisturizing and hydrating ingredients, and be sure to use products with sunscreens. A weekly mask or a hot oil treatment will keep chemically treated hair in good condition.

**Straight hair.** Choose a normal shampoo, because straight hair is usually in good condition unless it has been abused. Split ends and breakages are more noticeable in straight hair; a straightener or serum will help smooth.

**Fine hair.** Choose a volumizing shampoo, because fine hair tends to flatten and fly away. For styling, use mousse at the roots, add Velcro curlers at the base of head (in damp hair) and then dry. Also try a thickening agent or a dry shampoo when styling.

**Oily hair.** Use products that have jojoba oil (aids in removal of sebum, or hair oil), tea tree oil, rosemary and other nonabrasive cleansers. Dry shampoos or dry powders help fight oil.

**Thinning hair.** Aloe vera is soothing; neem oil, nettles and yucca stimulate the scalp; ginger, thyme and cayenne increase circulation; horsetail supplies calcium to the hair; and balm mint allows oxygen to flow into the bloodstream. Curetage® and The Morrocco Method® are a couple of natural brands that contain some of these beneficial ingredients.

> When hair is thinning, layers sometimes make it worse, with lost volume and flat hair. Instead, cut in a few short strands to add fullness when you backcomb (or you can perm or curl it).
>
> **BBG TIP**

## Black Celebrity Hair Hints

Grammy-nominated singer-songwriter Nicole C. Mullen uses a pH-balanced shampoo and alcohol-free conditioner. She also likes the Super Skinny® Serum by Paul Mitchell.

Actress Jada Pickett-Smith is a fan of Lisa's Hair Elixir and Hair Balm by Carol's Daughter®. Carol's Daughter is a brand created by Lisa Price and made without chemicals. Lisa likes to wear her hair natural without the use of blow dryers or irons, and one of her last steps in creating her natural 'do is applying a lightweight moisturizer, paying special attention to the ends of hair. Visit www.carolsdaughter.com to find out more about these fantastic products.

Ann Bruce, a writer, director and producer of stage and television, absolutely loves Trader Joe's Nourish Spa shampoo and conditioner. She has used many more expensive products, but really loves the affordable Trader Joe's brand. For deep conditioning, Ann likes ApHogee® Two-Minute Reconstructor followed by Queen Helene® Cholesterol Hair Conditioning Cream under a hair dryer. She alternates her ApHogee/Cholesteral regimen with AVEDA® Deep Penetrating Hair Revitalizer.

Ingredients to look for: shea butter, sea moss, rosemary, black vanilla, sweet almond oil, wheat germ oil and jojoba seed oil.

## Additional Hair-Care Products

There are products other than shampoo and conditioner that can help you maintain your hair in a healthy fashion. Here are a few of them:

**Leave-in conditioner.** Adds shine. Good for fine, flyaway or difficult hair. Apply away from roots to avoid an oily appearance.

**Serum.** Helps eliminate frizz. Usually also contains silicone, which gives hair shine.

**Hair mask.** Similar to everyday conditioners, but more concentrated (sometimes) with vitamins. Left on longer, it will penetrate the hair shaft. *Caution:* Don't leave on past the recommended time. After the mask is applied and distributed with a wide-tooth comb, cover or wrap your hair to lock in heat. End with a blast of cold water. Hair masks can be used once a week.

**Scalp care.** Take care of the skin beneath your hair with such products as Weleda® Rosemary Hair Oil or scalp elixirs from The Morrocco Method.

## THE RIGHT CUT AND STYLE

Hair care is only part of your 'do; now you need to decide what style suits you best. We all have different face shapes, lifestyles and personalities that will influence our preferred hairstyle. Take some time to evaluate if your style suits you, and if not, make a change.

Here are my basic guidelines for choosing a style to fit your face shape, but you and your stylist should discuss it.

### Determine Your Face Shape
- Stand in front of a mirror.
- Pull your hair back.

- Take an old lipstick or window marker and stretch at arm's length.
- Draw an outline of your face on the mirror and determine what shape your face most closely resembles: a heart, a square, a circle or oval/oblong.

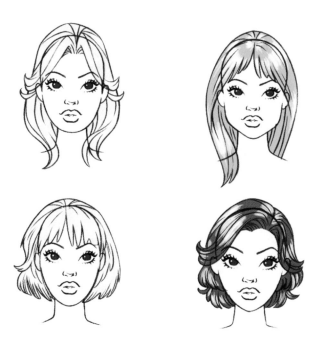

The following looks are best for these shapes:

**Heart.** Create height around the crown. Avoid a center part, which draws the eye to the chin. Graduated layers around face draw attention to eyes and cheekbones.

**Square.** Longer styles with soft layers soften the angles of the jawline.

**Round.** This would be me! Height at the crown gives a longer appearance, while layers cut along the side of the face give a more narrow look. At least shoulder length is best.

**Oval/Oblong.** Opt for bangs to shorten the face. Chin length adds width to the jawline.

A good haircut balances your face, head and body proportionately; fits your lifestyle; reflects your personality; and holds its shape for four to six weeks.

## Your Stylist

When you talk with her or him, make sure you understand each other. Before proceeding with a new hairstyle, ask your stylist these and similar questions: *Will this style be high maintenance? What is the upkeep for the color? Will there be a chemical reaction with my hair/scalp type? In your opinion, what is a good look for me?*

Remember: A style in a photo won't necessarily look the same on you as it does in the picture. Bring your photo to the stylist so that she or he can get an idea of what you like, but consider modifications she or he suggests based on your face shape, hair condition and hair type.

If you have trouble finding a stylist, ask your friends who have good haircuts. You can also look in the Yellow Pages or on the Internet for award-winning stylists or those voted "best in town." If you are on a tight budget, book a bang trim only; this will get you through another few weeks. Try your local cosmetology school for a cut or a blow dry. The instructor will be present and you will save money.

> **BBG TIP**
>
> A great website for trying out new hairstyles is www.thehairstyler.com. For a small fee, you can upload a picture of yourself and try on almost endless cuts and colors.

## CREATE CONFIDENCE WITH STYLE

Blow drying and styling your hair can be a difficult task, depending on your hair's texture. Every type of hair needs different styling products (these may include shampoo and conditioner, prestyle products and finishing products), tools (combs, brushes, blow dryers, irons) and time (how long you're willing to invest).

Shampoo and conditioner are important for your style, because they create the foundation. The right shampoo and conditioner can also help remedy many challenges you have with your hair: frizz, breakage, color fading, and so on. If you need volume in your style, use a volumizing shampoo and conditioner; if you need to add shine or softness to your hair, start with a smoothing and moisturizing shampoo and conditioner.

A prestyle product is any product used on wet hair to prepare it for blow drying. Again, depending on the style you want, use the proper prestyle product. For volume, you need a volumizing mousse and a root lifter. For shine and control, choose some type of shine serum and maybe a straightening crème. Be sure to ask your stylist what she or he recommends to achieve your style.

Once you have established a good foundation with your shampoo and conditioner and have prepared your hair, it's time to use your tools. Make sure you invest in a good blow dryer (see below for suggestions). They really are not all created equal. Weak dryers might take three times as long to get the job done, while some inexpensive models can get too hot and burn your hair.

> My stylist, Lulu, showed me how to achieve a quick style: Spray roots on the top of your head with volumizing spray. Part into sections and blow dry. Finish with shine serum, and let the bottom half of hair air dry.
>
> LULU TIP

Brushes are important as well. The right size brush will determine how much movement your hair has when it is dry. The bigger the round brush, the straighter your hair will be; the smaller the brush, the more movement, or curl, your hair will have. Paddle brushes are great for naturally straight hair that needs minimum smoothing and volume. A boar's hair or a tighter bristle brush won't brush through big sections of hair; it gives you maximum smoothing, but you have to work in very small sections. A metal or plastic bristle brush is easier to use, because you can work in bigger sections and achieve a smooth style.

Flat and curling irons take a little extra time but can really make a difference in your style. Make sure that when you use irons, you also use a leave-in conditioner and thermal protection, especially if you use them every day.

After you have spent time on your blow dry and style, you want to make sure all that work will last through the day! Finishing products can give you extra shine, volume, humidity protection, definition, hold, softness or texture. Shine sprays and glosses are a great way to finish long smooth and flowing hair. Hairsprays and waxes can help hold volume and style. Waxes and pomades create texture in all lengths of hair.

It used to be that I couldn't get my hair to look anything like Lulu, my stylist, could. That is, not until I had Lulu give me her secret for a great salon blow dry! You will love the fresh-from-the-salon results you get when you follow her step-by-step blow-dry basics.

1. *Remove dampness.* Once you've prepared your hair with the proper shampoo, conditioner and prestyle products, remove excess water by blow drying your hair every which way. If you start styling sopping wet hair, it will take you twice as long.

2. *Section your hair.* Depending on your hair's density, divide it into three to four sections to make it easier to control and save yourself time and frustration. Make one section across the nape, below the earlobes. Your next section should extend from there to the crown of your head, or you may divide that section in two down the middle, depending on the density of your hair. The last section is the horseshoe section on the top of your head.

3. *Give your hair smoothness and shine.* Starting with the back section, begin to blow dry, using your brush as an extension of your hand. Make sure you get enough heat on the ends of your hair to ensure maximum smoothing. Don't worry too much about heat damage, because you have already prepared your hair with a leave-in conditioner and a thermal protection. Once the first section is dry, go back over it until you are satisfied with the shine and smoothness. *When you think you've dried enough, dry some more.* A good amount of heat and brushing is what will give you salon-quality smoothness and shine. Move on to the

next section when you're ready. Since you've already sectioned your hair, all you have to do is remove a clip and drop the next section down.

4. *Give your hair movement.* If you want more of a bend or curl to your hair, use a smaller round brush on the ends. Hold the dryer on the ends as they are wrapped around the brush. Move the dryer back and forth across the brush to ensure that you don't keep the heat in one spot for too long. Once you achieve the curl or bend you want, move on to other sections.

5. *Give your hair volume and lift.* Once your back and sides are dry, you're ready for the top. For a more voluminous top, blow dry your roots in the opposite direction you want them to lie. In other words, up and forward, side to side. With that root lifter and mousse you used, it shouldn't be difficult to achieve. At the crown, blow dry roots forward and up. On the top sides, blow dry to the opposite side your hair will be lying. At the very top, blow dry forward. Once the roots are dry, direct the ends in the direction they need to go. You can finish your ends straight or with a curl or bend, depending on your style for the day. If you have a fringe (bangs), blow dry them side to side and then redirect the ends down, to the side, or however you wear them.

6. *Finish and lock in your style.* All that's left is to use the proper finishing product to keep your volume, shine, softness, texture or curl. This will keep your hair looking and feeling great all day.

If you need more hands-on help, ask your stylist to teach you the best and easiest ways to style your hair. A good stylist knows that if you can't duplicate your style at home, it's his or her job to teach you. Be patient and keep at it, and always use the products and tools your stylist recommends. Sometimes all you need is a little bit of practice and patience.

Laurent D, top hairstylist and native of France, has a long list of celebrity clients: Sharon Stone, Sophia Lauren, Terri Hatcher, Nicolette

Sheridan, Tea Leoni and Jewel, to name a few. Laurent has also put his signature mark on some of the fashion world's highest profile runways. I had the opportunity to interview the savvy hair designer and collect some insider tips on the stars as well as a few tricks of the style trade.

When we sat down, I asked Laurent, "What is Sophia Lauren like?" He smiled and described her professionalism, and said that she is a delight to be around. He told a story about how Sophia was once on set for a photo shoot and changed the lighting, after the photographer had spent two hours adjusting the equipment. With her eye for excellence, she knew what made her look best.

Laurent is also a great admirer of Tea Leoni, with whom he is raising money for breast cancer research. He has formulated Privé® Styling Brilliance for their cause, with portions of sales proceeds going to breast cancer awareness.

Laurent can style hair in 10 minutes, as he did mine. How? Blow dry (he uses brushes made by Mason Pearson®), part to the side, apply some product (shine serum, in my case), then use a curling iron or flat iron sporadically (he uses FHI® Heat Runway Ceramic Professional Iron). *Voilà!*

> **BBG TIP**
>
> Once hair is dry, tip it forward and give it a blast with cool air to seal the style.

I interviewed Christopher Hopkins, known as "The Makeover Guy," who has a passion for helping women look their best—and he really does a fabulous job! He has a great method for backcombing (for volume) in his awesome book, *Staging Your Comeback: A Complete Beauty Revival for Women Over 45*:

1. Take small sections (one inch) and pull taut straight up from the scalp.

2. Using the back of a teasing comb or a fine-toothed comb, push the hair to form a matte as close to the scalp as possible. Start at the very base and build up; do not start pressing hair at mid-

shaft or higher, or the matte will not be at the scalp but will be floating in the middle of the hair shaft.

3. Continue with small sections where you want the volume.

4. Spray hairspray (lightly) and allow to dry.

5. Comb over the foundation with a fine-toothed brush or comb, style hair, and spray.[1]

Hair in the summertime should not be too straight; it should be loose and flowing. Finish with fixable hair spray.

## TOOLS OF THE TRADE

The last thing we want after washing and styling our hair is to end up with the frizzies. Whether straight or curly, short or long, our hair can be smoother with a few tools of the trade.

### Hair Dryers: Invest in the Best!

- **T3® Tourmaline Featherweight Dryer.** Why is it good? Dries 60-percent faster than other hair dryers, weighs only 13 ounces and generates the most negative ions/infrared heat. Warning: It's a bit pricy.

- **T3 Tourmaline Overnight Dryer.** Try this option for a lower cost.

- **Parlux® 3200 Ceramic Ionic Dryer.** A stylist favorite.

- **Conair® Professional Tourmaline Ceramic Ionic Styler.** A great choice for a good deal.

### Irons

Curling and flat irons are great styling tools, but which ones work best? I personally use irons made by CHI®, but any iron with infrared, ions or

ceramic will help take out frizz. Good quality models are made by FHI®
and Corioliss®, while Hot Tools® makes less expensive irons that work
fairly well. Visit www.misikko.com and www.sortprice.com for closeout
deals on these brands. Because great hair tools can be pricey, pick your battles when it comes time to purchase them. Rank your list from "most
wanted" at the bottom to "must have" at the top.

Be sure not to abuse irons; from time to time, give your hair a rest.
The only time I blow dry is when I have a special event, and I wash my
hair two to three times a week to avoid too much heat.

## Diffusers

These attach to the nozzle of a blow dryer and are good for creating
wavier hair or making curly hair tighter. Diffusers also help to defrizz. You
can find one to fit most any hair dryer at retailers that carry hair styling
appliances.

## Rollers

Using rollers for a quick style can bring waves to straight hair or smooth
out curls.

### Velcro Rollers

Use on dry hair, set with hairspray and heat with blow dryer. Give a
minute or so to cool then tease or back comb.

### Hot Rollers

Tuck in the ends of your hair neatly and remove curlers when cool.

## Brushes and Combs

Use the right kind of brush or comb for smooth styling:

- Round ceramic curling brushes create bounce.
- Vented paddles give a smooth finish and are good for
  longer hair.
- Wide-tooth combs are perfect for wet hair, whether after
  showering or when applying leave-in conditioner.

- Tail combs are used to section hair or create the perfect part.
- Pick combs separate curls without frizzing curly hair.

## Styling Products

**Gel.** Sculpts and styles your hair. Water-soluble resins and silicones provide a firm hold. Apply to wet or damp hair.

**Mousse.** Light and airy product that allows for even distribution. Usually gives a lift and hold depending on the strength and ingredients. Apply at scalp and root area when hair is damp.

**Wax.** Gives shine and holds strands with an adhesive consistency. Good for short hair or to give ends a sharp look. Use after blow dry.

**Styling crème.** Protects hair from heat; moisturizes hair and leaves it soft and silky. Great on curly hair, colored hair or straightened hair. Apply when hair is damp.

**Serum or shine enhancers.** Creates shine, often due to silicone. These products can make hair dryer over time, and too much will make your hair appear oily. Use on dry or wet hair.

**Straightening balm.** Closes down the cuticle to achieve a smooth and sleek finish. Apply to wet hair, then blow dry.

> Make your own hair gel. Mix 2 tbsp. of flax seeds and 1 cup of water in a saucepan and bring to a boil. Remove from heat for 15 minutes, and then strain. Add a few drops of your choice of essential oil, then pour mixture into a storage container. Keep uncovered until mixture thickens, then seal tightly.
>
> **BBG TIP**

## HAIR COLOR

Proverbs 16:31 says that "gray hair is a crown of splendor," but we're going to color anyway! (Only if you want to!) Gray hair is typically a result of natural aging. Pigment (called melanin) in the hair shaft comes from special cells at the root of the hair. These cells are genetically programmed to make a certain amount of melanin at specific ages. At some point in the aging process, these cells make less and less melanin until the hair has very little pigment. White hair has no pigment, and gray hair has much less than red, black or brown.

Some women use color to cover gray, while some use color for a new look. If you choose to color, it's best to do so every four to six weeks and be consistent with the product and shade. Some hair dyes can be toxic, so make sure you read the next chapter, "The Devil's Top-10 Ingredients" to find out what brands to avoid.

John Masters is an amazing stylist who has a green salon in New York. He uses only the best nontoxic colors around (he has a product line called John Masters Organics that includes moisturizers, shampoos and conditioners and is fabulous). When I spoke with John, he told me that in his salon, he uses Herb UK's Organic Color System and Elumen hair color made by Goldwell. (Elumen is the first oxidant-free durable hair color that works without peroxide or ammonia. Negatively charged color is drawn deep inside positively charged hair and is held, as if by a magnet, through entirely natural processes.) John also said that for home color, he likes Herbatint Herbal Hair Color Gel, one of the cleanest on the market. Henna is also a good choice, but doesn't cover gray hair as well.

John's tip for softening hair at home and giving extra shine: Mix the juice of one whole lemon with five to six ounces of apple cider vinegar. Pour mixture over your head and comb through to ends. Leave mixture on for 10 to 15 minutes and rinse.

## NO MORE BAD HAIR DAYS

No woman wants to leave the house having a "bad hair day." With a little time and the right products for your hair, the forecast for your hairstyle will be great. You'll feel that your hair looks its best and suits your personality, mood and agenda. We all want to look our best, yet still keep the right perspective on our God-given beauty. If you follow the hair-care guidelines in this chapter, you'll check that mirror before you leave the house with a smile at the beautiful, unique woman God created!

Here are a few last-minute tips:

**Bad hair day.** If your styling efforts are going nowhere, why not create a trendy ponytail? Place your pony low, closer to your neckline, for a classic style. Accent your ponytail with a bandanna or a pretty barrette.

**Roots.** Eye shadow or brow shadow is a great fix for when you can't make it to the salon or color your own hair. Use a shadow brush to sweep matching color onto roots. Mineral powders stay on best, or try a mascara. *If you dare:* Create highlights with gold mascara, which rinses right out the next time you wash.

**Dirty hair.** No time to wash? Try a dry shampoo (Ojon® makes one called Rub-Out™ that has been well reviewed) or a baby wipe when oil builds up. You can also dab facial toner over your scalp with a cotton ball.

**Frizz alert.** My friend Celia shares her easy-smoothing secret: Before you enter the shower, wrap a bandana around your head and cover with a shower cap. The heat of the shower will activate the natural oils in your hair. Presto! No frizz.

# Six

# The Devil's Top-10 Ingredients

May I have some formaldehyde, topped with ethyl acetate and imidazolidinyl urea, with a side order of butylated hydroxytoluene sprinkled with phthalates, please? Oops, I forgot to ask for bleached napkins."

You may think, *I'd never eat something so toxic.* But if you use many of the cosmetic products available at the corner drugstore, your skin consumes it every day. Skin is not like plastic, sealed up tight against toxins; it's more like a sponge, soaking up everything you put on it. Products that go *on* our body are as important as what goes *into* our body. You may be eating healthier, but do you pay attention to what you put on your face and hair? And what you use to clean your house? Ingredients in many of these products are toxic.

This chapter is not meant to scare you but to help you understand that the government, which regulates the ingredients in personal care and cleaning products, isn't always looking for the healthy option. You need to be your own researcher, get the magnifying glass out and become a label detective. It's imperative to learn some ways to avoid toxicity. I named this chapter "The Devil's Top-10 Ingredients" but I have to tell you that there are way more than 10 out there; we are living in a chemical soup, from our environment right down to the safe haven of our homes. Since

World War II, more than 80,000 synthetic chemicals have been introduced to our society; "production rates for synthetic petrochemicals have burgeoned from 1 billion pounds per year in 1940 to over 400 billion pounds per year in the 1980's [imagine what it is now!]."[1] Many of these chemicals are in our food supply, skincare, cleaning products and lawn care, affecting our health and the health of our planet.

Have you ever wondered why your skin gets irritated or your throat gets a little sore or you have nasal burning sensations after using certain cleaning products? Chemicals trigger inflammatory responses, which we recognize as heat, swelling and redness. This occurs in the tissues of your face, in your arteries and in your vital organs when your immune system is under attack. The more poisons you are exposed to, the more inflamed your body becomes.

If such harsh ingredients are toxic to humans, why do companies use them? Because they can. The cosmetics industry remains largely unregulated, unlike food and drugs. In America, nine chemicals are banned from personal care products, while in the European Union, more than 1,100 chemicals are banned because they may cause cancer, birth defects or reproductive problems. Another reason synthetic ingredients are often included is that they cost a fraction of their natural counterparts, making them attractive to manufacturers.

According to Charlotte Vohtz, a pharmacologist and founder of the organic Green People Company, "Most women absorb around two kilograms [more than four pounds] of chemicals through cosmetic products every year." She explains how:

> Scientists have shown that chemicals in cosmetics can pass through the skin, into the bloodstream and internal organs. Oily solutions such as moisturizer and foundation are designed to be absorbed. Lipstick is swallowed, and both eye shadow and mascara can be absorbed by the mucous membranes.[2]

In 2004, the Environmental Working Group evaluated ingredients in 7,500 personal-care products for safety. Here's what the EWG discovered:

- One of every 120 products on the market contains ingredients certified for use by government authorities yet known as probable human carcinogens, including shampoos, lotions, makeup, foundations and lip balms.

- Seventy-one hair dye products contain ingredients derived from carcinogenic coal tar.

- Fifty-five percent of all products assessed contain penetration enhancers, ingredients that can increase a product's penetration through the skin and into the bloodstream, increasing consumer exposures to other ingredients. Fifty of these products also contain penetration enhancers in combination with known or probable human carcinogens. Nearly 70 percent of all products contain ingredients that can be contaminated with impurities linked to cancer and other health problems.

- Fifty-four products violate recommendation for safe use set by the industry's self-regulating cosmetic ingredient review (CIR) board.

- Nearly all products (99.6 percent) contain one or more ingredients never assessed for potential for health impacts by the CIR.

- For more than half of the ingredients approved by the CIR, "the panel fails in whole to discuss any available data with respect to cancer and mutagenicity, birth defects, and other reproductive risks."[3]

## HIDDEN DANGERS IN THE POWDER PUFF

### 1. Talc

Let's consider a well-known ingredient found in a ton of food, makeup, skincare, powders and medicine products: talc. What is talc? According to the Cancer Prevention Coalition, "Talc is a mineral, produced by the mining of talc rocks and then processed by crushing, drying, and milling. Processing eliminates a number of trace minerals from the talc, but does not separate minute fibers which are very similar to asbestos."[4]

You may be thinking, *Talc has been around for years, so how can it be dangerous?* Talc particles have been shown as the cause of tumors in the ovaries and lungs of cancer patients. Because of these findings, in 1973, the U.S. Food and Drug Administration (FDA) drafted a resolution that would limit the amount of asbestos-like fibers in cosmetic-grade talc. According to the Cancer Prevention Coalition, no ruling has yet been made. More than 25 years later, cosmetic-grade talc remains unregulated by the federal government.

Your best bet is to stay away from talc and try other alternatives, such as mineral powders, cornstarch or rice powder for oil absorption.

## 2. Coal Tar

Coal tar, often found in eye shadow, is also linked to cancer. Lipstick can contain high levels of artificial colorings made from coal tar derivatives, which can cause allergic reactions. Lead, which is poisonous to humans, is also sometimes found in lipsticks; check www.ewg.com to find out the percentage of lead found in your brand of lipstick. Color additives certified by the Federal Food, Drug and Cosmetic Act (FD&C) are often made from coal tar, too.

## 3. Nitrosamine

This preservative is often used in foundation, cured meats and pesticides, and pollutes water and air. Some epidemiological studies have associated increased incidence of human cancer with the presence of nitrosamine.

## 4. Formaldehyde

Yes, the same stuff that preserves deceased bodies is used in makeup, bubble bath, shampoo, conditioner, moisturizers, and a whole lot more. Sodium lauryl sulfate, an ingredient often used in detergents and personal-care products, may contain formaldehyde as a preservative, and other toiletries may have it without listing it on the label. For instance, imidazolidinyl urea and DMDM hydantoin may release formaldehyde that can cause migraines, allergies and asthma.

## 5. 1,4-Dioxane

This petroleum-derived carcinogenic compound is used intentionally in drycleaning solvents, lacquers and automotive coolant. Yet dioxane also shows up in personal-care products because it is the byproduct of some manufacturing processes, including the process by which sodium lauryl sulfate becomes sodium laureth sulfate. Dioxane is a known animal carcinogen and probable human carcinogen, as well as a skin and lung irritant. It is strongly suspected to be toxic to the kidneys and nervous system. It appears on California's Proposition 65 list of substances known to cause cancer or birth defects.

Although dioxane can be vacuumed-stripped out of personal-care products for pennies, this step is often not taken by manufacturers. And because it shows up in many sudsing products, an individual may be exposed multiple times each day through different products.

Since it is an impurity, not an intentional ingredient, dioxane does not appear on ingredient labels. For consumers, that means going one step further to avoid products containing petrochemical ingredients that often come along with dioxane contamination. These include the ingredients or partial ingredient names: "PEG," "polyethylene," "polyethylene glycol," "polyoxyethylene," the suffix "-eth" (such as sodium laureth sulfate), "oxynol," "ceteareth" and "oleth."[5]

## 6. Parabens

Paraben preservatives were developed in the 1930s to stabilize crèmes, and are now used in nearly all skincare products. Yet recently, researchers have discovered a possible connection between parabens and both breast cancer and male reproductive problems. While these findings are disputed by some scientists, many others, including the European Scientific Committee on Consumer Products (SCCP) have determined that parabens cannot be ruled safe in personal care products.[6]

So why do some "companies for women" allow such toxic ingredients in their products and at the same time support breast cancer awareness and host fundraising walks for breast cancer research and education? Most of the ingredients these manufacturing companies use in their products are unsafe and untested, yet they still co-opt the pink ribbon. I am happy they want to raise money for the cause, but perhaps they need to take some of that money and invest it in safer, more natural ingredients.

## 7. Triclosan

Found in antibacterial products such as deodorant soaps, vaginal deodorant sprays, toothpastes, mouthwashes and sanitizing hand gels, as well as household cleaning products, there is some concern that triclosan may negatively affect both the endocrine and the nervous systems. It also lingers in ground water and sediment to have an impact on the environment. According to a comprehensive study conducted by the University of Michigan School of Public Health, plain soaps are just as effective as antibacterial soaps, and do not pose the same health risks.[8]

*f you're still not convinced about the importance of avoiding parabens, check out this brief Q&A with Dr. Gloria Gilbére:*

❧ *Why should we use paraben-free products?* Because anything that can "clog" the system adds to our toxic total body burden.

❧ *Can synthetic products get into our liver?* Absolutely. Everything we put on our skin gets absorbed throughout our body. The liver's function is to neutralize. If we're "dumping" toxic ingredients into our liver faster than its ability to neutralize, disorders and illnesses will emerge.[7]

## 8. MSG

Most famous as an ingredient in Chinese food, monosodium glutamate lurks not only in your food, hidden under alias names, but also in your personal-care products. MSG is a neurotoxin and affects the brain directly. Repeated exposure can lead to Alzheimer's disease, depression, skin rashes, asthma attacks, epilepsy and behavior problems.[9] Some common ingredients that contain MSG are: hydrolyzed proteins, amino acids, yeast extracts, glutamic acid, glutamates and naiad. For a complete list of hidden MSG-related names, check out truthinlabeling.org/hiddensources.html.

## 9. Phthalates

Think of the potent aroma of a vinyl curtain or that new car smell. You're smelling phthalates. Pronounced THA-lates and produced in the amount of 1 billion tons per year, phthalates hold scent and color in a variety of products. Phthalates are a group of man-made chemicals that are structurally related to phthalic acid, which is organic. The most important use of phthalates is in plastics, especially PVC, where they act as plasticizers. Phthalates are also present in a wide range of industrial, household and consumer products (including personal-care products), such as pipes, vinyl wall and floor coverings, roofing materials, safety glass, car parts, lubricating oils, detergents, food packaging, adhesives, paints, inks, medical tubing, blood bags, pharmaceuticals, footwear, electrical cables, stationery, nail polish, hair sprays, soaps, shampoos, perfumes, moisturizers and (until recently) toys.[10]

Earl Gray, a top phthalate researcher at the U.S. Environmental Protection Agency, has said that phthalates disrupt the production of testosterone, which is critical for the masculinization of the male species.[11]

## 10. Triethanolamine (TEA)

TEA, if combined with nitrosating agents such as 2-bromo, 2-nitro-propane or 1,3-diol, becomes carcinogenic. On its own, TEA is a skin sensitizer and is possibly toxic to the lungs and brains. The Material Safety Data Sheet on TEA says, "Hazardous in case of skin contact, of eye contact, of ingestion, of inhalation."[12] It is commonly found in floor polish, pool cleaners, rug cleaners, laundry detergent and toilet bowl cleaners, in addition to cosmetics.

## NATURAL VS. SYNTHETIC: BECOME A LABEL DETECTIVE

Now that we've dissected a few of the ingredients to avoid, you may think, *Well, as long as I look for "natural" products, I should be okay.* Not so fast! The word "natural" can be misleading. As you read product labels to determine ingredients, the following definitions of "natural" and "synthetic" may be helpful:

- *Natural* suggests that the ingredients are derived from natural sources rather than being produced synthetically. However, there are no industry standards demanding that "natural" products contain *all* natural ingredients. A few natural ingredients may be added to a synthetic product or a product may have no natural ingredients at all, and still be labeled "natural." The word "organic" can also be deceiving, as we discussed in an earlier chapter. Look for "USDA Organic" and the seal of certification.

- *Synthetic* indicates a substance that is the result of a chemical process that does not occur in nature. This process begins with naturally occurring plant, animal or mineral sources, but is manipulated in a lab to produce a new substance not found in nature.

Now you need to become a label detective. You've likely been reading food labels in the grocery store already, but now you must decipher the labels of your personal-care products as well.

Before you begin, you must know that ingredients are listed in order of the total percentage they make up of the product, with the highest percentage first. It is a legal requirement that all skincare products must be labeled with ingredients in descending order of their quantity. According to

In Stacy Malkan's book, *Not Just a Pretty Face,* she lists the chemical ingredients of products she commonly used on a daily basis:

✿ 22 daily doses of parabens, along with four other suspected hormone disrupting chemicals

✿ 17 hits of chemicals with limited or mixed evidence of carcinogenicity. One ingredient, petroleum distillates in my Cover Girl Marathon Waterproof Mascara, is banned in the European Union.

✿ 17 applications of penetration enhancers, which can draw the other chemicals more deeply into my body

✿ 15 doses of chemicals that persist in the body or accumulate up the food chain

Narelle Chenery, director of research and development for Miessence®
Certified Organic Skin, Hair, Body and Health Products, a good rule of
thumb is to divide the ingredients list into thirds. The top third usually
contains 90 to 95 percent of the product, the middle third usually contains
5 to 8 percent, and the bottom third contains 1 to 3 percent.[15]

Let's take a look at a real label and dissect it:

---

**Product: Apricot Cream**

*Ingredients: Natural or organic ingredients include:*

1. Water
2. Isopropyl palmitate (palm oil derivative)
3. Apricot kernel oil
4. BIS-diglyceryl caprylate/caprate/isostearate/stearate/hydroxystearate adipate (vegetable triglyceride)
5. Glyceryl stearate SE (vegetable-derived)
6. Caprylic/capric triglyceride (glycerin-derived emollient)
7. Ceteareth-12 (organic emulsifier)
8. Tocopherol oil (vitamin E)
9. Chamomile extract
10. Sage extract
11. Linden extract
12. Balm mint extract
13. Shea butter (from karite)
14. Wheat germ oil
15. Carrot oil
16. Cetyl alcohol (organic co-emulsifier)
17. Sodium hydroxide (pH adjuster)
18. Sorbic acid (organic compound)
19. Tocopherol acetate (vitamin E derivative)
20. Methylparaben (organic compound)
21. Propylparaben (organic compound)
22. Imidazolidinyl urea (organic compound)
23. Fragrance
24. FD&C Yellow No. 5, D&C Red No. 33.

*Content: Apricot oil (2.5% [out of 100%])*

---

- ❧ 15 products with fragrance—an unspecified mix of chemicals likely to contain phthalates and allergens
- ❧ Less than half the ingredients in my products have been assessed for safety.[13]

When she tallied them all up, Stacy could not believe what she was putting on her body.
She wondered about the two benign lumps that had required surgical removal and about
her four-year struggle with infertility. Could her health issues be due to the fact that, in
addition to the chemicals in her personal-care products, Stacy lived a mile away from the
largest polluting trash-burning facility in her state? "In the real world, my lungs breathe
the air from the smokestacks and the fumes from the rug cleaner at the same time my
skin absorbs the toxic chemicals from the face lotion."[14]

About 90 percent of this product is water and isopropyl palmitate, which is made from isopropyl alcohol, synthetic alcohol and palmatic acid, a fatty acid derived from palm oil. Isopropyl palmitate is known to cause skin irritations and dermatitis in rabbits and has been shown to have comedogenic properties (that is, it causes acne).[16]

Ingredient numbers 4, 5 and 6 are all produced by chemical reactions between various fatty acids and glycerol (synthetic glycerine), and can cause allergies and dermatitis. Number 7 is a synthetic emulsifier that can contain levels of etylene oxide and dioxane, both of which can be harmful. Numbers 8 to15 are natural ingredients used in very small amounts that may have been grown using pesticides. Number 16 may be natural or synthetic and has been shown to cause contact eczema. Number 17 is otherwise known as "casutic soda," and is alkaline, corrosive, and inhalation causes lung damage (the FDA banned use of more than 10 percent in household liquid drain cleaners). Number 18 was once made from the mountain ash berry but now is commonly made from a synthetic preservative—not so natural. Number 19 is synthetic vitamin E, made in a lab. Numbers 20 to 22 are toxic and allergenic preservatives. Number 23 may be synthetic and can contain phthalates. Number 24 is synthetic color.[17]

Most cosmetics have one or more of the following, either natural or synthetic: emollients, humectants, emulsifiers, surfactants and/or preservatives. Let's take a look at the function of each of these, and consider a few natural alternatives.

**Emollients** serve two functions: They prevent dryness and protect the skin, acting as a barrier and a healing agent.
- *Synthetic*: PEG, synthetic alcohols, hydrocarbons
- *Natural alternatives*: cocoa, shea and jojoba butters, plant oils (avocado, rosehip), honey

**Humectants** keep the skin moist.
- *Synthetic*: propylene glycol, ethylene/diethylene glycol, synthetic alcohols
- *Natural alternatives*: lecithin, panthenol (pro-vitamin B5), glycerin

**Emulsifiers** hold two ingredients together that normally don't mix.

* *Synthetic*: alkoxylated amides (TEA, DEA, MEA), PEG compounds

* *Natural alternatives*: plant waxes (candelilla, carnauba, jojoba, rice bran), xanthan gum, quince seed

**Surfactants** are substances capable of dissolving oils and holding dirt in suspension so that they can be rinsed away with water.

* *Synthetic*: sodium or ammonium lauryl or laureth sulfate, TEA, DEA, MEA, PEG

* *Natural alternatives*: castile soap, yucca extract, soapwort, quillaja bark extract (some can be coconut-derived)

**Preservatives** extend the life of the product. Synthetic preservatives are often used because they are cheaper and last longer than natural alternatives.

* *Synthetic*: imidiazolidinyl urea (Germal 115) and diazolidinyl urea (Germal 2), parabens

* *Natural alternatives*: tea tree oil, thyme essential oil, grapefruit seed extract, D-alpha tocopherol acetate (vitamin E)

Understanding ingredients and decoding what they really are will allow you to be consumer savvy. Yet many products do not list ingredients directly on the package; so where can you find the information? Call the company or look on their corporate website. You can also find information from consumer sites, such as databases of Material Safety Data Sheets (try www.hazard.com/msds), the Environmental Working Group (www.ewg.org) and the Environmental Protection Agency (www.epa.gov). Also check out *The Safe Shopper's Bible: A Consumer's Guide to Nontoxic Household Products, Cosmetics, and Food* by David Steinman and Samuel S. Epstein; *A Consumer's Dictionary of Cosmetic Ingredients: Complete Information About the Harmful and Desirable Ingredients Found in Cosmetics and Cosmeceuticals* by Ruth Winter; *Not Just a Pretty Face: The Ugly Side of the Beauty Industry* by Stacy Malkan; and *Pure Skin: Organic Beauty Basics* by Barbara Close.

## THE BEST INGREDIENTS: GOD'S

We can't let the devil have the last word! Next time you shop for cosmetics and household cleaners, look for healthier alternatives. God's ingredients are better for you and better for the environment. When we buy and prepare foods closer to the way God made them, we are healthier. The same can be said for other products.

Unfortunately, sometimes in Christian circles, being "green" or being friendly to the environment is looked at with suspicion. Yet Adam was in charge of his environment, the Garden of Eden; you could say he was the first tree hugger (see Gen. 2:15)! Like Adam, we should be good stewards of all God has entrusted us with.

I recently met Peter Illyn, a Christian environmentalist with Restoring Eden, a ministry that is "dedicated to encouraging faithful stewardship of the natural world as a biblical, moral, and wise value."[18] I was so pleased when I read this statement on the organization's website: "Restoring Eden's mission is to make hearts bigger, hands dirtier, and voices stronger by re-discovering our biblical call to 'speak out for those that cannot speak for themselves' (Proverbs 31:8) as advocates for wild habitats, native species, and indigenous culture. . . . We are Bible-believing Christians who strive to walk in justice, mercy, humility, and other-mindedness."[19]

We all need to take responsibility for our planet and ourselves, from our homes to our bodies and to the homes of animals and plants in the wild. We are in this together; God made it that way. Contributing to the health of our environment helps humans and wildlife, and it preserves our world for our children and grandchildren to come.

Until recently, most of us have been shopping in the dark. But now we are turning on the lights to see product labels; we're finding out exactly what is going in and on our skin and our earth. Here are some ways we all can benefit, not just in what we buy, but in how we live each day:

1. BYOB—Bring your own bag next time you shop.
2. BYOB—Bring your own bottle of water.
3. Turn off the lights when you leave the room. (My dad used to say, "I'm not J. Paul Getty. Turn off those lights!")

4. Take shorter showers.

5. Eat more veggies. (Locally grown is better; locate a farm or farmer's market near you at www.localharvest.org.)

6. Cancel delivery of your phone book; we almost all use the Internet now anyway.

7. Sign up for online banking and cancel your paper statements.

8. Eat what's in season; it costs a lot more to ship and buy out-of-season produce.

9. Use natural, not artificial, fragrances.

10. Buy something vintage.

11. Switch to rechargeable batteries.

12. Use a power strip, and when you're done, turn it off.

13. Change your light bulbs from incandescent to compact fluorescent.

14. Run a full load of dishes—more dishes, less water-intensive hand washing.

15. Carpool.

16. Buy greener cosmetics.

17. Wash your clothes on "Cold."

18. Look for the greenest drycleaner or the best household cleaner at www.greenmaven.com.

*Beauty in balance means a healthier you.*

19. Go for bamboo (from flooring to cutting boards).

20. Join a food co-op.

21. Drive 55 mph and inflate your tires properly to save gas.

22. Get a library card.

23. Buy fair trade imports.

24. Buy organic pet food.

25. Use a natural alternative for lawn pest control.

Do the best you can, and don't let others make you feel guilty. If you can't afford certain products, organic clothing or organic foods, find alternate ways to make smarter, healthier choices. Ask God to show you a plan for how to live a healthier life; He knows your heart, and He will show you the way. Beauty, health and our environment go hand in hand. It's about balance.

# Seven

# The Pampered Pantry

Sitting at the kitchen table, enjoying a fresh-brewed cup of coffee, I hear my husband come in. He whispers, "Good morning," and sneaks a kiss. Suddenly, spitting coffee grounds, he exclaims, "What is on your face?!"

"Well, honey, you told me to slow down on the spending, so I decided to turn our kitchen into a spa. Welcome to Shelly's Pampered Pantry, where the food tastes good and your wife looks good, too! Doesn't my coffee mask taste, I mean, *look* great? Well, the results will, and they won't cost you a penny."

You may think, *How crazy is that?* But trust me: Your face and body—not to mention your pocketbook—will thank you when you turn your kitchen into a spa. Here are some home recipes that will beautify with ingredients you probably already have on hand. Open the fridge and let the beauty treatments begin!

## PAMPERED PANTRY 101: NO COOKING REQUIRED

### The Continental Breakfast Beauty Treatment

Would you believe that applying warm, used coffee grounds will tighten up your face? The caffeine in the coffee stimulates and energizes tired skin.

Leave on for one minute, and then rinse clean. Hop into an empty tub with the remaining grounds and rub them all over your skin. Wait 10 minutes, fill the tub with warm water and take a coffee-bath break. Your thighs will thank you for their smooth appearance. When you get out of the tub, mix one teaspoon of lemon juice in one cup of water, saturate a cotton ball, and apply to your face. This will remove any residue and shrink your pores.

Another mask choice is plain, unsweetened yogurt. To tighten pores and cleanse, spread plain yogurt over your face, wait 20 minutes, and then rinse clean with lukewarm water. Or, before taking a shower, cover your entire body with plain yogurt and layer with olive oil. Wait 10 minutes, then rinse clean. Dry off and spread any remaining yogurt on a bagel and enjoy with a fresh cup of coffee.

> **BBG TIP**
>
> Put home spa ingredients in a muffin tin and use as a tray while in the bathroom or kitchen. You might also put a tin in a drawer for use as a desk or makeup organizer.

## The Baby Aisle

How about some Pantry ideas for eliminating dark circles, making pimples disappear and cleaning your hair (without washing)? It all starts with a visit to the baby aisle of your grocery store! *Warning*: If you don't have an infant, your husband may freak out when he sees some of these items:

1. A jar of baby food bananas
2. Burt's Bees Diaper Rash Ointment
3. Seventh Generation® Chlorine-Free Baby Wipes

Women are all about multi-tasking, so if your baby has a rash and you have a pimple, here's a simple solution to both problems: Put rash cream on his tush and dab some on your blemish. The zinc in the cream heals, dries and takes the red out of both irritations.

If you don't have time to wash your hair, use a baby wipe on the roots for an instant hair revival.

Finally, spread the contents of a 6-ounce jar of bananas over clean skin under your eyes. Wait 10 minutes and then rinse clean. The potassium will help eliminate dark circles (whether from sleep deprivation caused by caring for a fussy baby and husband or by working late on that big report).

## Whiter Nails and Kissable Lips

Are your fingernails or toenails looking yellow? Dissolve two Efferdent® denture-cleaning tablets in a bowl of water, and then soak your fingers and/or toes in the solution for five minutes. Your nails will come out whiter, just like the commercial promises for dentures! Dab your nails with lip balm and buff.

Do your lips need to be rejuvenated? Apply non-petroleum jelly to dry lips, then use an old tooth brush to gently exfoliate away dead skin.

> Use an Efferdent tablet in the mug you forgot to rinse out; it will remove coffee or tea stains.

**BBG TIP**

## Quick Relief for Tired Feet

Grab a salad or mixing bowl and mix a solution of warm water, white vinegar and lemon juice. Soak your feet for 10 minutes and then rinse. Pat dry and apply coconut oil (a great moisturizer) to cracked or dry feet. File and buff toenails with lip balm. There's no need to polish because vinegar removes stains and lemon juice works as a whitener and tightener.

Let's sum up:

*A day at the spa = $400*
*A day in the Pampered Pantry = $5*
*Your husband not yelling when the credit card*
*bill arrives = Priceless*

# PAMPERED PANTRY 102: RECIPES FOR RADIANCE

Now that you've completed the prerequisites, you're ready for more advanced fun!

## The Formula for Great Skincare

As we have seen, many companies make skincare product lines with synthetic ingredients and then pass them off as "natural." Don't fall for it! Read the label; chances are that if you can't pronounce it, you don't want it on your skin. If you haven't been able to find reasonably priced skincare products made with *real* ingredients, why not consider making your own? Step into your kitchen/Pampered Pantry/lab and create revitalizing skincare formulas. I want instant results without going bankrupt. If you're like me, here are some skin remedies that will remap lines, tighten pores and bring new life to your beautiful face the natural way . . . and the *affordable* way.

### The Wrinkle Remapper

Orange oil revitalizes skin, while almond oil replenishes moisture. (Not recommended for sensitive skin.)

- 8 drops sweet orange essential oil
- 1 teaspoon almond oil
- 2 teaspoons hazelnut oil

*Combine ingredients. Use two fingers from one hand to hold skin taut and the other index finger to massage wrinkle area. With daily application, wrinkles will soften.*

### Line Reversal Mask

Rose oil calms irritated skin, softens wrinkles and relaxes the central nervous system. Almonds are a natural emollient and honey hydrates.

- 5 drops rose oil
- 2 teaspoons almond oil
- 2 tablespoons honey

*Mix together and apply to face and neck with fingers. Relax for 15 minutes, and then rinse with warm water. Pat dry.*

> Create index cards with skincare recipes and file under "Natural Beauty" in your recipe box. As you plan meals, don't forget to include your skin's "food list" when you buy the rest of the groceries.
>
> **BBG TIP**

### Tighten and Revitalize

Chickpea flour is an effective skin-softening exfoliant; it stimulates circulation and rebuilds tissue. Bananas, known as a source of potassium and vitamin A, help reduce redness and puffiness. Eggs tighten pores and leave your skin renewed.

- 4 tablespoons chickpea flour
- 1 ripe banana
- 1 egg, beaten

*Blend first two ingredients in a bowl, then add beaten egg. Apply mixture to face and neck. Leave on for 15 minutes, then rinse well with warm water. Pat dry.*

### City Slicker Mask (for oily skin)

Does your skin feel like there was an oil spill on the bridge of your nose? This mask is the cleaner-upper of all slickness! Cucumbers are a mild astringent known for anti-inflammatory properties that can relieve skin irritation, smooth roughness and heal abrasions. The egg white tightens, lemon cuts the oil and mint is an antiseptic.

- $1/2$ cucumber (skin on)
- 1 egg white
- 1 tablespoon lemon juice
- 1 teaspoon mint

*Puree ingredients in a blender and refrigerate for 10 minutes. Apply the mixture to your face and leave on for 15 minutes. Rinse with hot, then cool water. Pat dry.*

*Papaya Enzyme Mask*

The enzymes in papaya fight free-radical damage and are known to reduce age spots and fine lines for a natural facelift. Oatmeal exfoliates, binds the skin and moisturizes; its cellulose and fiber mean more elastic skin. Honey contains vitamins, minerals and amino acids to nourish skin (and hair).

- 1 tablespoon honey
- 1 papaya, peeled and seeded
- 1 tablespoon oatmeal (ground in coffee grinder or food processor)
- 1 teaspoon lemon juice

*Blend papaya, then pour into a bowl and add remaining ingredients. Apply mask to your face and leave on for 20 minutes. Rinse with warm water. Pat dry.*

*Georgia Jewel Mask*

My grandmother's name is Georgia Jewel Long. She's from Tennessee, not Georgia, but she loves Georgia peaches *and* smoother skin. Peaches are high in antioxidants and skin-softening enzymes, while egg white tightens skin and reduces the appearance of large pores.

- 1 peach, pitted
- 1 egg white

*Puree peach in a blender. Beat egg white until stiff, and then fold peach puree into the egg white. Apply thick layer to face and neck with fingertips. Let dry 15 to 20 minutes, then rinse with lukewarm water. Pat dry.*

## Personalized Powders

### Dusting Powder

| | |
|---|---|
| 8 ounces tapioca starch | 4 ounces arrowroot powder |
| 4 ounces corn starch | 14 drops grapefruit oil |
| 7 drops ylang-ylang oil | |

*Combine powders and mix well. Apply oils to absorbent cotton pad. Place oiled pad in container with powder, shake or stir well and allow to sit 24 hours. Shake or stir well and allow to sit another 24 hours. Shake or stir well, remove pad and discard. Place powder into powder box, and it is ready to use. Makes 2 cups.*

## Light Dusting Powder

11 ounces tapioca starch
1 ounce kaolin powder

4 ounces baking soda
15 to 18 drops jasmine or vanilla oils

*Combine powders and mix well. Apply oils to absorbent cotton pad. Place oiled pad in container with powder, shake or stir well and allow to sit 24 hours. Shake or stir well and allow to sit another 24 hours. Shake or stir well, remove pad and discard. Place powder into powder box, and it is ready to use. Makes 2 cups.*

## Fabulous Feet

## Brown Sugar Foot Scrub

2 tablespoons brown sugar
2 tablespoons aloe vera gel
1 teaspoon freshly squeezed
lemon juice

2 tablespoons ground oatmeal
(ground in coffee grinder or food processor)
1 tablespoon honey
1 teaspoon almond or olive oil

*Mix all the ingredients in a large bowl until it resembles a paste. Use circular motion and massage gently into heels, arches, toes and ankles. Rinse with warm water.*

## Refreshing Foot Powder

$1/2$ cup cornstarch
$1/2$ cup rice flour
1 teaspoon powdered ginger
10 drops lavender oil

$1/2$ cup oatmeal flour
$1/2$ cup powdered arrowroot
10 drops tea tree oil

*Combine powders and mix well. Apply oils to absorbent cotton pad. Place oiled pad in container with powder, shake or stir well and allow to sit 24 hours. Shake or stir well and allow to sit another 24 hours. Shake or stir well, remove pad and discard. Place powder into powder box, and it is ready to use. Makes 2 cups.*

# CREATE A DO-IT-YOURSELF-AT-HOME SPA PARTY

A day at the spa is costly, going by yourself is not the most fun and finding a babysitter is another job in itself. Why not do it all at home? Oh, yes! You'll have a blast creating the theme for the party and getting your kids involved, too!

I decided to do a beach theme because we live in Florida. To keep my kids busy, I had them design decorations—fish, seagulls, anything to do with the ocean—while I worked on other preparations. The Oriental Trading Company has loads of party stuff for every theme, and it's inexpensive, so you can buy most of the decorations and goody bag items through them. You can be simple or go all out, depending on your budget. I bought hibiscus straws for drinks, themed cups, fish tattoos for the kids, plastic leis, hibiscus picks for finger food and a burlap table runner. (The price for everything came to $18.95 plus shipping.)

For my guest list, I stuck with eight women. To lighten the load and price, I had each friend bring one of the fixings for the facial bar. (For instance, one person brought five avocados, while another brought a large container of yogurt.) I also asked each person to bring one toiletry to contribute to a giveaway gift bag.

### Menu

Peach Zinger and Finger Foods
Facial
Pedicure
Dessert and Tea

## Welcome!

I welcomed my guests with finger foods and peach zingers. These delicious smoothies are made with fresh or frozen peaches, cinnamon, almond milk, ginseng and cloves, and they spice everyone up from the start. I chose a playlist of ocean sounds, instrumental Hawaiian music and the soundtrack from *Finding Nemo*. In the next room, I covered the furniture with bedsheets and set up supplies for finger-painting and face-painting. (I also made sure there were plenty of healthy goodies to eat!) I asked one of the older kids to supervise the activities, and had a kid-friendly movie ready for emergencies.

## Facial Bar

Transform your dining room or living room into the "facial fixings" section, where your guests will mix their own beauty treatments.

*Pick the Fixings*

Fill clear glasses or Jell-O glasses with a variety of exfoliants and astringents. I chose oats, yogurt, smashed avocado, honey, grapeseed oil, lemons, crushed green tea leaves and essential oils such as peppermint, lavender and rosemary.

*Set the Bar*

Put out a tray of the above ingredients. On a separate tray, arrange empty glasses and stirrers (such as Popsicle sticks) for mixing. Also include cotton swabs, cotton balls and moisturizer. Have paper towels handy and cotton face towels nearby.

*Do Your Facial!*

1. Cleanse
2. Choose and mix your mask
3. Apply and leave on for 15 minutes
4. Rinse and pat dry
5. Apply toner and moisturizer

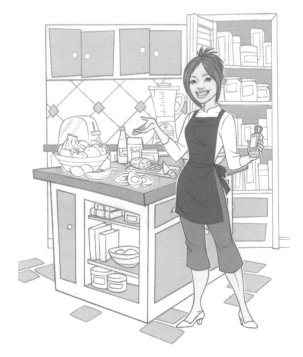

### Mask Ideas to Inspire Your Creative Juices

- $1/2$ cup oatmeal, 2 tablespoons honey and $1/4$ cup plain yogurt; mix into paste, apply and leave on for 15 minutes.
- Mix 1 avocado and 4 tablespoons yogurt; spread and leave on for 30 minutes.
- Avocado eye mask: 5 drops almond oil and $1/2$ avocado; blend, apply around eyes and leave on for 5 minutes.
- Mix $1/2$ cup yogurt, 2 tablespoons tea leaves, $1/2$ teaspoon lemon; apply and leave on for 15 minutes.

Be creative—anything goes. A cool website called www.recipegold mine.com has a ton of masks to choose from.

If you want to add some treatments, try massaging problem areas before applying your mask. Depending on your skin type, mix your own essential oil with a carrier. For instance, try:

*Oily skin*: 1 ounce hazelnut oil, 6 drops rosemary oil and 4 drops lemon oil

*Sensitive or dry skin*: 1 ounce hazelnut oil, 6 drops rosemary oil and 4 drops lavender oil

*Normal skin*: 1 ounce hazelnut or grapeseed oil, 6 drops lavender oil and 4 drops rosemary oil

## Foot Treatments

### Relaxing Foot Soak

Now for those tired feet, invite your guests to the pedicure bar, where they can enjoy a relaxing soak. Most of the ingredients for this fabulous soak are already in your pantry:

| | | |
|---|---|---|
| 1 teaspoon honey | $1/2$ cup coconut milk | $1/4$ cup Epsom salt |
| 1 sprig rosemary | 2 ounces olive oil | $1/2$ cup cornmeal |

*In a small bowl, mix ingredients. Pour into a foot bath (or salad bowl!) filled with hot water. Soak feet for a few minutes. Using undissolved mixture, exfoliate rough spots.*

Invigorating Leg Rub

*After rinsing, mix 1/2 cup almond or soy oil with 4 drops peppermint oil. Massage into feet and legs to refresh tired legs.*

*Have another tray filled with nail polishes, polish remover and nail files. Paint each other's toenails (or splurge and hire a nail tech from a nearby cosmetology school).*

## Guilt-Free Dessert

Top the spa experience off with cookies and tea—try tulsi or rooibos teas; the antioxidant benefits are wonderful.

---

### Orange-Pecan Cookies

1 cup chopped pecans
1 teaspoon grated orange zest
1 egg white, lightly beaten
Powdered sugar

$1/3$ cup sugar
1 teaspoon orange extract
Canola-oil cooking spray

*In a food processor, pulse pecans and sugar into a sand-like texture. Transfer to a mixing bowl and stir in orange zest and extract. Slowly stir in egg white until a thin dough forms. Cover and chill at least 2 hours. Heat oven to 350 degrees. Lightly coat a baking sheet with cooking spray. Divide dough into 16 heaping teaspoons and roll each into a ball. Place balls 2 inches apart on baking sheet. Bake 8 to 10 minutes. Cool and dust with powdered sugar.*

---

## Gift Bag Giveaway

Put the guests' toiletry items into a gift bag, top off with a tiny soy candle and draw one guest's name from a hat. You'll send one blessed girl off with a glow!

There are so many spa party themes to choose from: Thai, Moroccan, Mexican . . . just about any culture or country. Even a Royal Spa Party would be great—you could serve High Tea wearing an avocado mask and a big floppy hat! Spa parties will work well for special occasions such as bridal or baby showers and birthday parties, and every woman in your church would love a Mother's Day spa party. Have a Girls' Night In (and what about the men?). The list is endless . . .

Or have a party of one, just you. Indulge yourself in a milk bath or a relaxing mask while you read the book you haven't had time to pick up in three weeks. Take time out for you; schedule an hour in your planner for "me" time. We are better wives, mothers and daughters when we relax and take time to get our thoughts together. We need regular breaks to be of good service to others.

What better way to lift your spirits than by taking care of you. Release, relieve and be renewed!

# Eight

# Clothing Essentials for Potential

"I have nothing to wear!" How often have you said this? You can learn to make the most of what you have, to maximize the clothes that give you confidence, and to avoid style disasters by dressing appropriately . . . all without breaking the budget.

What we wear tells others a lot about us. It's an extension of who we are. When we dress with confidence, we exude God's beauty. That's why it is so important to dress appropriately. When you pick clothes off the clearance-aisle rack, consider more than just the price tag and that it's an "Oprah favorite." Do your homework: Evaluate your body type, as well as the colors and the styles that flatter your shape, before you invest in your "modest but hottest" wardrobe. You don't have to lose your style; you just have to make it work for you. Be creative!

## KNOW YOUR BODY SHAPE

The real secret of knowing how to dress is becoming more aware of your body's assets and challenges. Start with knowing your body shape. Below are five basic body types and what to avoid when dressing each. The general rule is finding and maintaining balance based on your shape and size.

## Circle or Apple

This shape, as the name implies, carries weight in the midsection. You have larger breasts, narrow hips and thinner or shapely legs.

### Pants

Choose pants that have flatter pockets in the front, zippers on the side or the back side. Opt for tailored pants, trousers should fit loosely (not baggy) and pants or jeans with a slight flare in the leg. Avoid low-rise jeans; they will reveal too many curves.

### Skirts

A-line skirts and circle skirts that cling to the waist before flowing to just above the knee will emphasize the appearance of hips.

### Tops

Wrap-around tops create the illusion of a waist. Empire and V-necklines are also flattering.

### Shoes

Wedges and pointy-toed heels will give height, while small kitten heels are always cute.

## Triangle or Pear

This shape carries more weight in the hips and thighs and is narrower in the chest and waist.

### Pants

Choose straight-leg or boot-cut pants or jeans that have a slight flare toward the hem. Mid-rise jeans will make your hips look smaller.

### Skirts

Opt for straight, dark-colored skirts that are tapered near the hemline, A-line skirts or wrap skirts. Pencil skirts with vertical seams are also slimming.

### Tops

Wear shirts with wide lapels, cowl neck sweaters or shirts with square necklines that will broaden the shoulders.

*Shoes*

Ankle straps or chunky heels can weigh you down; try peep-toe heels instead.

## Cone

You carry weight at the top, in your chest and/or shoulders, and the goal is to balance your shape by visually widening the hips and upper legs.

*Pants*

Wider-leg pants will add fullness where you need it. Choose flared-leg pants or jeans; boot-cut adds volume mid-length to create balance.

*Skirts*

Likewise, flared skirts add balance to the legs; a pleated skirt that hits right at the knee will do the same. Avoid pencil skirts, which will make your hips look too small.

*Tops*

Pick empire tops, tailored dress shirts and V-necks to give proportion. Don't wear halter tops, which will make your arms and chest look larger.

*Shoes*

Chunky heels and platforms are a good choice to give weight on the bottom.

## Rectangle

This shape is straight bottom to top with few curves, more of a "boy shape" with not as much of a waistline.

*Pants*

Semi-fitted pants or jeans paired with a long-length top will bypass the waistline.

*Skirts*

Choose A-line, circle and trumpet skirts that hug your waist, then flare out slightly toward the hemline to give contour to your waist. A shirt dress or other dresses that fit loosely through the waistline would be good choices.

## *Tops*

Try a long jacket, or layer jackets and tops to create interest. Wear a tunic that falls loosely to the high hip, with V-neck and U-neck. Try a wrap top as well.

## *Shoes*

Avoid chunky heels; they will make you look bottom-heavy. Try pointy-toe heels instead.

## Hourglass

You have a full bottom and medium-broad shoulders, with a defined waistline. You don't really have to make up a balance, as you already have one.

## *Pants*

Most stylists recommend straight-leg jeans (though I have an hourglass body shape and wear jeans that have a little flare in the leg . . . I like to live dangerously!). Choose jeans that have full-size back pockets so that your rear doesn't look too big. Opt for creased or vertical-striped pants.

## *Skirts*

Tailored skirts are nice hemmed right at the knee, and A-line skirts work well, too.

## *Tops*

You'll look great in open-neck wraps, tailored shirts and fitted tops (empire shirts are not the most flattering, but I do own a couple). Limit yourself on crew- and turtlenecks, and peasant tops shouldn't be your first choice, either.

## KNOW YOUR BEST COLORS

How can you learn what colors work best on you? One place to start is to recognize what color you're wearing when you receive the most compliments. Then consider the following three things together to determine your best color schemes:

- **Hair color.** With hair color and wardrobe, the goal is to complement without clashing. (For example, if you are a redhead, oranges and reds that complement your hair may be difficult to find; likewise, yellows and creams if you are blonde. Opt for contrasting colors instead.) If you have medium or ashy hair color, use your wardrobe to brighten up; if you have brassy or vivid hair color, choose clothing that won't conflict with your bold look.

- **Skin color.** Are you warm-toned, cool-toned or neutral-toned? You can do a quick test to find out. Buy some foil wrapping paper in gold (warm) and silver (cool). Hold a piece of foil below your chin and look in a mirror to see which hue enhances your natural glow, then build your wardrobe around warm (golden) or cool (silvery) tones. Neutral tones fall between the extremes of blue and yellow. If this describes you, opt for hues that bring out your eye color instead of your skin.

- **Eye color.** If the eyes are the windows to the soul, the curtains should complement them! Your wardrobe should bring out your eyes. For instance, if you have green eyes, wear more and varying colors of green to accent them. Play up your eyes—they can be your best asset.

When I talked with Brenda Kinsel, author of *Brenda Kinsel's Fashion Makeover: 30 Days to Diva Style!*, she suggested talking to a friend or hairdresser about what colors complement you if you can't see for yourself in the mirror. In her book, Brenda includes fill-in-the-blank spaces for your hair color, skin tone and eye color. When you've written them down, she says to go to your closet and see if you have colors that echo those you listed.

Don't toss out all your clothes in the wrong colors; just wear the right color closer to your face, or from the waist up. Experiment with colors and color combinations to find the right ones for you.

In *Fashion Makover,* Brenda suggests these great color combinations:

*Warm and Spicy*: raspberry/turmeric, lentil/spruce, raspberry/
nutmeg
*Cool and Natural*: cool gray/soft blue, lavender/slate blue
*Light and Spirited*: kiwi/tomato, wheat/tomato
*Royal and Opulence*: black/golden yellow, emerald/purple
*Organic and Botanical*: acorn/oak, olive/sesame
*Feminine and Classic*: soft pink/deep wine, dusty
amethyst/berry[1]

Unless you're a politician or a talk-show host, it's best to go with neutral colors (black, gray, earth tones, white, cream) for suits and main clothing pieces, with spots of color to brighten your ensemble. A good guideline is at least half of your wardrobe made up of solid (some pinstripes are okay) neutral colors.

For further research, check out the resources in the appendix, or, if you can afford one, contact a color consultant.

The following colors and shapes can instantly slim the appearance of your body:

- Black, charcoal, navy and chocolate brown. Darker colors slim you, while lighter colors make you appear bigger.
- Monochromatic dressing is more slimming.
- Tailored cuts, not tight clothing.

Have you tried SPANX® body shapers? They drop you a size instantly, and you can find them just about anywhere. My friend LeAnn could not believe how she got into the tiny slimmer, but she was even more stunned at how trim she looked.

## SHOPPING FOR CLOTHES

Keep your body shape and color in mind as guidelines for creating a wardrobe that "fits" who you are and what you do. When shopping, look for quality, not quantity; be skeptical about trends; and dress for your age, but with your own personal flair.

## Find Your Personal Style

Your personality and how you spend your time (as a stay-at-home mom, at a corporate job, volunteering) should help determine your personal style. Whether your style is corporate and classic, bohemian and creative, bold and dramatic, or soft and romantic, it needs to fit you.

Look through magazines to give you inspiration. Some of my favorite style icons are from the past, such as Jackie Onassis and Audrey Hepburn, and their style has influenced my favorites from today, such as Anne Hathaway. I see what I like in a magazine and then put my own twist on it . . . and you can, too. Even if the outfit on a certain person is too revealing, I take what I like and make it modest.

## Go Green and Go Vintage

I had the pleasure of talking to the Vintage Queen herself: Allison Houtte, author of *Alligators, Old Mink & New Money: One Woman's Adventures in Vintage Clothing*. She also owns a store in Brooklyn, New York, called Hooti Couture. Allison is a beautiful woman inside and out; she giggles when customers tell her that she should model (she has graced the cover of *Vogue* and other couture magazines).

I asked Allison what to look for when going vintage, and she gave me the scoop:

**BBG:** *What should you look for when buying vintage clothing?*

**AH:** Not so much names . . . you need to love it. Go with what your style is and don't pay top dollar.

**BBG:** *What is your best buy?*

**AH:** I found a Pucci suit at a church sale. It was gorgeous! Velvet two-piece for five dollars!

**BBG:** *Name your favorite hot spot when you buy vintage.*

**AH:** "Flamingo" in Miami and thrift stores in Key Largo.

**BBG:** *When buying fur, what should one look for?*

**AH:** Definitely look for—and avoid—dryness and shedding. Give it a good shake. If it's shedding, put it right back down. And if the skin is cracked or the fur feels a little rough when you try it on, or if it doesn't give, then keep moving.

**BBG:** *Do certain types of fur last longer than others?*

**AH:** Mink is a more durable fur. Rabbit is beautiful, but rips and sheds easily. When you're into vintage fur, the big thing is chinchilla. They're hard to find, but once you touch chinchilla, you never go back. Also, don't forget fake furs. Because faux fur doesn't dry up or rot the way real fur can, it can pretty much last forever.

**BBG:** *What do you do if you're having a stressful day?*

**AH:** Jump into the shower, wash your hair. When you get out, go put something pretty on that makes you feel good. Put on some lipstick and a Barry White CD.[2]

A cashmere cardigan from the 1950s . . . a velvet evening coat . . . a silk scarf by Pucci, Lanvin or Courreges . . . two faux leopard coats, in '50s trench and '70s swing . . . a vintage watch from the '40s . . . a 1920s crystal broach . . . finding them may take some time and commitment, but these treasures will be gorgeous additions to any wardrobe.

## When and Where to Shop

Some of my favorite stores are Macy's, Dillard's, Off 5th (the Saks Fifth Avenue outlet), T J Maxx, Ross, Marshalls, Arden B., Mango, Caché and Bloomingdales (sales only!). I sometimes find good deals at Ann Taylor Loft, Old Navy, The Gap, TopShop.com, LaRedoute.com, Target, Asos.com, Steve & Barry's, Kohls, Beltz and JC Penny.

For great deals, shop in August for summer items, November for fall, February for winter and May for spring (especially Memorial Day weekend). Other sale days include December/January, the Fourth of July, President's Day and Labor Day.

## Create a Style Guide

Be your own stylist! A great way to keep a great style is to put together out-fits and then take photos. For example: Place a blouse, pants, blazer, hand-bag, shoes and jewelry together on your bed; mix and match until you're happy with the whole look. Then take a picture and put the photo in an album called "Beauty by God Style System," or whatever title you choose. Be creative with your notebook—I bought a scrapbook on sale for half-off at Michaels Arts and Crafts Store and enjoy the artistic side of keeping it up to date as much as the practical side.

Categorize your threads by season, then group them by events such as "work," "dinner out," "outdoor" and "indoor party," "wedding," "PTA meeting," and so on. (Women also occasionally need a special outfit for when we feel a little bloated; include a picture of an outfit that is comfort-able for that time.)

In the front of your style notebook, have the names and numbers of your hairstylist, esthetician, dermatologist, makeup artist (even if she is at the cosmetics counter), shopping buddies and drycleaner/seamstress (also include backups!). Have one pocket for coupons and pictures to add, and another for your "want" list and outfit ideas. With everything in one place, you can take your notebook along the next time you go shopping. You'll know exactly what you're looking for, and will be less likely to im-pulse buy or overspend (and your hus-band will be thrilled!).

## Finding the Perfect Pair of Jeans

No matter what your size or shape, I bet there have been times when you've been tempted to believe that "the perfect pair of jeans" is a myth, much like "the Easter Bunny" or "comfortable stilettos." I'm here to tell you that the perfect pair of jeans is not just a fairy tale, and that you can track them down if you follow these simple guidelines:

1. **Length**. First, decide whether you'll be wearing these jeans with heels or flats. If the jeans are too long and you wear flats, the bottom hem will tear. If you are taller, Victoria's Secret carries jeans with inseams from 30" to 36". Alloy (Alloy.com) has a 37" jean that is budget-friendly. The Gap, Lucky Brand, Silver (Silver Jeans.com) and Ann Taylor also make jeans with longer inseams.

2. **Rise**. Depending on your body shape, choose where you want the waistband to sit. If you have lovehandles, opt for a rise that sits *over* rather than under—no muffin tops, please!

3. **Fit**. "Stretch" and "Relaxed" are user-friendly and comfortable. "Slim" and "Lean" are more tight-fitting.

4. **Cut**. Slightly flared-leg jeans are universally flattering, but especially good for medium to tall women. More petite frames also look great in straight-leg or tapered cuts.

5. **Waist**. A contoured waist, that starts higher on your behind and dips lower in front, is best (avoid "plumber crack," ladies!). You should be able to fit two fingers between the waistband and your skin—any pair of jeans that inhibits respiration does not qualify as "perfect"!

If you're plus-sized, look for larger rivets, bigger pockets and over-sized buttons. One friend of mine loves Apple Bottoms® jeans; she swears that their signature large pockets shrink even the plumpest rear. Be sure back pockets are placed near the center; if they are too far apart, your tush will appear wider. If your bottom is flat, opt for pockets that have a button or a fold-over to give the appearance of fullness.

If most of your weight is on the bottom, keep your eyes open for boot-cut dark denim in a low rise, and pair with an eye-catching top to draw eyes up. Side seams that wrap forward give legs a leaner look, and lighter shades emphasize . . . so avoid stone-washed on problem areas. If you want to "unfade" your jeans instead of tossing them, try a dye. While there are currently not very many organic fabric dyes on the market, at least you're using what you have instead of throwing your jeans

away to purchase another pair. A classic denim shade is made by Dylon®
(find it at Chaffinch.com). After you have dyed your jeans, soak them in
a textile softener such as Milsoft (Dharmatrading.com) because dyeing
can harden fabric.

My favorite jeans are Citizens of Humanity, but I just bought an organic pair made by 7 For All Mankind on sale at Nordstrom. Here are
some of my friends' favorites:

"Rock and Republic, Seven Jeans, Juicy Couture (on sale) . . .
really, it's the fit." —*Tammy Trent, recording artist and author*

"Rock and Republic, and Citizens of Humanity."
—*Candace Cameron Bure, actress*

"The sweetheart jeans by Old Navy because they fit my hips, but
aren't too baggy around my waist. The key to finding a pair of excellent fitting jeans is to look for jeans with a bit of a span-
dex/lycra content (no more than 5%) because the jean will stretch
to fit your body." —*Kathryn Finney, author of* How to Be a
Budget Fashionista: The Ultimate Guide to Looking Fabulous
for Less

"Banana Republic, hands down." —*Anita Renfroe, author
and comedienne*

"I rarely wear jeans but when I do, I like one pair of skinny jeans
and they are from The Gap, believe it or not. They always make
me feel skinny and they help when I feel like fitting in with everyone else and not being so severely individualistic." —*Danielle
Kimmey, recording artist (Out of Eden) and speaker*

"I wear Ann Taylor because of the length. Most stores don't have
long inseam, so go online—the inseam is up to 37 inches."
—*LeAnn Weiss-Rupard, author*

## Shoes, Shoes and More Shoes (and Bags, Too!)

How many is too many? I'm not going to tell you how many I have. My
excuse is that it's hard to find the right fit *and* the right look. I really don't

like shoe shopping—I'd rather shop for jeans—but I have found a couple of stores that I can get out of in less than four hours (sort of kidding). DSW has great deals on cute shoes (they also carry men's). I like the bargain section. You can also find good quality for reasonable prices at T J Max, Ross, Macy's and Dillards.

Some basic colors and styles to keep on hand: sling-back heels, peep-toes, boots and sandals (make sure your toenails look neat), in classic black leather. Neutral colors such as beige, khaki and cream go with a variety of outfits (if you're a little more daring, try metallic gold or silver). Printed pumps are cute, too—just avoid busy pants.

**BBG TIP**

Has your heart ever felt like it wanted to jump out of your chest when you slipped on a slick floor? Try Heart Stoppers™ to keep it from happening again! These heart-shaped no-slip shoe pads stick to the soles of your shoes for a sturdy step, every time.

While we're on the topic of great accessories: I love handbags. They can make or break an outfit. I know it's tempting, especially if you're a mother, to carry a purse big enough to hold a Bentley. But do you really need a bag that's bigger than you? Reevaluate the surplus supplies in your purse, and consider downsizing. Your back and shoulders will thank you.

Some cute bags are made by Nine West, AboutAttitude (adorable and inexpensive), Chinese Laundry and ShopSueyBoutique.com. Check out Macy's and Dillards for great sales on bags.

Let me make a confession: I have walked the streets of New York's Chinatown and gone into the back room to buy a fake Chanel, Louis Vuitton or Christian Dior handbag. But not long ago, I began to hear that the sale of counterfeits is connected to child labor, drug trafficking and even terrorism (I gave up the fake bags). Counterfeiting costs American businesses up to $250 billion annually and is responsible for the loss of more than 750,000 jobs in the United States.[3] To learn more about fake fashion, visit www.fakesareneverinfashion.com or www.myauthentics.com.

## Our Cups Runneth Over

Are you a victim of spillage from the top and sides? You may need to get measured for a new bra size, which is easy to do at Nordstrom or Macy's. As we get older, our bra size changes; we can't expect to wear the same size as in college, especially after having kids. The right-sized bra will allow you to feel more comfortable and will make your blouses look much nicer (no back bulge or muffin top).

Wearing a lacy bra under a T-shirt will make you look lumpy. Instead, try the T-Shirt Bra™ by Bali. I got my T-shirt bra at Macy's on sale (of course); it's made without wire by Warner's.

> Larger bustlines should avoid tops with ruffles.

**BBG TIP**

If you are a larger bust size, try Wacoal or Playtex brands. DKNY, Fantasie™ (at select Nordstroms) or Cacique™ (Lane Bryant) are great if you need a lift. Need to banish back bulge? SPANX Brallelujah™ is made with no wires.

## Eco-Chic

I am so happy to see more mainstream brands going organic or environmentally conscious. For so long, eco-friendly fashion has been extremely expensive, but it is becoming more and more competitive. Banana Republic tags its Green Collection with an iconic elephant, while Target is partnering with designers focused on organic fabrics. JC Penney's Arizona® brand for men makes recycled T-shirts, jeans and cotton shirts and shorts. More brands, such as Levi's and Josephine Chaus (Sam's Club), and more stores are carrying organic clothing. Check the Resources section at the end of this book for online eco-shopping tips.

## MODESTY IS THE BEST POLICY

The Bible says to "leave and cleave," not "leave and cleavage!" Dress with modesty in mind so that our brothers' minds don't go wild. Think about how you look.

What does modesty look like? Below is an excerpt from an article I wrote for the fine arts issue of *On Course* magazine. It was intended as a set of guidelines for young women on worship teams, but I think these tips are a good place for all of us to start, whether on or off the stage.

- *The "Praise and Raise" Test.* Looking in the mirror, raise your hands. Is your midriff showing? If so, choose a longer shirt.

- *The Trampoline Test.* If more than your hair bounces when you walk onstage, you may need a more supportive undergarment or a looser shirt. Push your top against your chest bone; if the fabric bounces back quickly, your top is too tight.

- *Prevent mini disasters.* Skirt hems should be at or below the knee—the longer the better, depending on stage height.

- *Consider your coif.* The saying, "The higher the hair, the closer to God," isn't true onstage. Your 'do can be fun, but keep it neat.

- *Tank-tops are a no-no.*

- *Avoid the painted-on look.* Can you pinch an inch of your jeans or pants on the thigh area? If not, they are too tight.

- *Don't wear pajamas.* If the top you are wearing looks like it should be concealed under clothing (i.e., camisoles), keep it covered up.

Modesty means observing the proprieties of dress and behavior; it doesn't mean you can't be creative! Here are some ideas to help you express the style that is uniquely you:

- **Accessory Savvy.** Accessorize to maximize. Try some strappy sandals, wedges or loafers. Wear scarves, belts, barrettes, bandanas, headbands and jewelry.

- **Layered Look.** Layer colorful tops and bright tunics over slim pants or jeans, cardigans over tank-tops, and vests or jackets over shirts.

- **Lifted Hands.** Have clean, manicured nails. Remember, the J-Factor is something that should be visible whether you are on or off the stage. We represent Christ and should always strive to glorify Him. At the end of the day, the best outfit you can wear is confidence.[4]

For one reason or another, some women get upset about this modesty thing. Not too long ago, the male employees of a rather large Christian company raised some concerns about the women's outfits; they felt that their female colleagues' clothing choices were too revealing. In response to the complaints, one of the VPs of the company had a women-only meeting that featured a fashion show of modest and appropriate attire. This did not sit well with the ladies; in fact, the presentation backfired a bit. Instead of the women putting their brothers' spiritual wellbeing above their own preferences and convenience, they treated the men as if they were pigs.

For her book *For Women Only*, Shaunti Feldhahn interviewed a group of randomly selected Christian men.[5] The ones who were married reported devotion to their wives. Shaunti proposed a hypothetical situation in which an attractive female colleague gives a presentation, and asked the men what they might be thinking as they watched her talk up front. Here are a few of their answers:

- "Great body . . . stop it! What am I thinking?"
- "I check to see if she's wearing a wedding ring."
- "I wonder if she finds me attractive."
- "I bet she uses those curves to sell this deal."
- "I wonder what's under that nice suit? Stop it. Concentrate on the presentation."
- "About two minutes into her talk, I'd be remembering a scene from a porn video I saw when I was fifteen."

Men are wired differently than women. This does not make them evil. It does not make them animals. It just makes them different. There is some evidence that about 25 percent of women are stimulated visually, but that is a low percentage compared to the vast majority of men who are turned on by what they see. No, I don't think women should walk around in ankle-length, A-line skirts and a veil (though I can understand the appeal, at times). I am saying that if we look in the mirror and think, *Maybe this is too revealing*, it most likely is.

When in doubt, do the three-point check:

- **Bend over:** Can you see "the sisters"? If so, wear a tank-top under your shirt.

- **Butt check:** Can you see your underwear lines or thong silhouette? Switch to boy shorts (try Barelythere.com) or SPANX.

- **Breast silhouette:** Look in the mirror; are your breasts completely contoured? If so, your shirt is too tight; go up one size.

I know this may seem extreme for some of you, but remember: God made men, and we have to keep them around if we want to procreate. We'll just have to forgive them for being born that way. (I am so kidding . . . I had to put that in there for my husband, who has eyes only for me: 20/20 "Shelly Vision.")

Do you remember the terrific sister group Out of Eden? Danielle Kimmey was one of the trio, and is now a part of The Revolve Tour. Danielle says that she didn't used to care about modesty; she never saw anything wrong with her wardrobe until her sisters would point certain things out to her. Now, at 27, she has grown some. She says that "our bodies are the temple of the Holy Ghost, and they need to be protected . . . when the sexy comes into your wardrobe, you've gone too far . . . we have a responsibility to ourselves."[6]

## CLOSET INTERVENTION

Now that you know what to wear and how to wear it, the next step is to check out what you already have. Examine your closet to find the treasures and toss out what you don't need or shouldn't wear. Have a friend help. This mini-questionnaire will help you evaluate the staples in your closet.

## Choose Your Top Three

*The top three outfits I wear are:*

1. _____

2. _____

3. _____

*The top three jewelry pieces I wear are:*

1. _____

2. _____

3. _____

## Ask Yourself

*The colors others compliment me about most are:*

1. _____

2. _____

3. _____

*The colors I feel great in are:*

1. _____

2. _____

3. _____

*My close friends compliment me most when I wear:*

1. _____

2. _____

3. _____

*My favorite trends are:*

1. _____

2. _____

3. _____

*Some clothes I've always wanted to buy, but never have are:*

1. _____

2. _____

3. _____

## Use It or Lose It

| | | |
|---|---|---|
| Do you love it? | Yes____ | No____ |
| Have you worn it in the last three years? (Some people might say in the last year, but I think there are some timeless pieces in our closets that deserve to be kept, such as a black velvet gown or trench coat.) | Yes____ | No____ |
| Is it still in style? | Yes____ | No____ |
| Is it in good condition (e.g., fibers are not worn down from too many visits to the drycleaners)? | Yes____ | No____ |
| Does it flatter your body? | Yes____ | No____ |
| Is it comfortable to wear? | Yes____ | No____ |
| Did your husband or grandmother buy it and you feel too guilty to toss it? | Yes____ | No____ |

**BBG TIP**

If you really love that favorite skirt, bring it to a good seamstress along with new fabric and have it cloned.

## Edit Your Closet

Separate your apparel into these five categories. Remember, sometimes you have to be ruthless!

1. Trash it!
2. Give it! (Business attire can be donated to www.dressfor success.com, The Salvation Army or a local church.)
3. Alter it!
4. Clean it!
5. Get it out next season!

## Organize Your Clothes

- **Upgrade your hangers.** Toss out the wires (actually, recycle them to the drycleaner) and replace them with plastic or wooden (try Huggable Hangers® from the Home Shopping Network, www.hsn.com).

- **Group similar items.** Skirts with skirts, pants with pants, long and short sleeve tops, and camisoles by color and fabric. When your garments are streamlined, you'll want to wear them.

- **Hang up your shoes.** Shoes should be stored on slanted racks or in a hanging bag, not on the floor where dust can settle on them. You can also keep them in their original boxes. (Place a photo of the shoe on the outside of the box.)

- **Belts to the back.** Belts may be placed on individual hooks on the back wall to prevent belt buckles from scratching each other. This also makes your selections easier to see.

- **Shelve your bags.** Bags should be placed upright on shelves to help them keep their shape.

- **Dress up your closet.** Add boutique touches by painting the walls a vibrant shade, installing a crystal pendant lamp or by accessorizing with white wicker or vintage pieces. Get inspired and make a collage of clothes you would love to wear.

## Coordinate by Season

If space is limited (no extra closets), try plastic containers, pretty boxes from your favorite store or even a boot box (wrap it in your favorite colored paper) to store clothes until you need them. Include a sachet of lavender oil to keep away moths and musty smells. When stowing winter or summer garments, be sure to have all items cleaned before you put them away.

Keep your sweaters folded on your top shelf between wire separators or baskets (lay tissue paper down so that material does not snag), or place them in a storage container under the bed. Hang heavy blazers and winter outfits in another closet (or under the bed in storage containers).

## Tricks for Preserving Your Garments

- **Steamer/iron.** I use one by Rowenta® at home, and travel with a model made by Jiffy®. Instead of drycleaning your clothes after one wear, give them a rest and steam them. It will save you money and your clothes from harsh chemicals.

- **Sweater dryer.** This is a mesh platform for drying knits and hand-wash items. Laying them flat to dry will help them keep their shape and last longer.

- **Fabric shaver.** This handy tool glides over clothing to remove lint and pills. For delicates, use a velvet lint brush.

- **OxiClean® for whites.** Avoid drycleaning white shirts, which can turn yellow over time from cleaning chemicals. Hand wash or machine wash delicates. Use OxiClean to wash, then iron yourself or take to the cleaners for steaming.

**BBG TIP**

When you pick up your clothes from the drycleaner, remove plastic immediately and hang garments outside for several hours before moving to the closet. This gives chemicals time to evaporate and reduces health risks. Also check out www.nodryclean.com or www.findco2.com for safer drycleaning options.

## Fashion Emergency Kit

Have you ever worn a red shirt under a cream jacket and then looked like you sweat red? I was so mad when my jacket came back from the drycleaner and the red sweat was still there! I wish I had used a nifty little invention called Garment Guard™. These are disposable, self-adhesive cotton disks that adhere to the inside of your clothing, creating a barrier between your underarm and your garment. No more sweat rings!

Here are a few more gadgets that can save you time and money. Include them in a "fashion emergency kit" that you tuck away in case of a crisis.

- **Strap Tamers™.** Tame savage, stubborn bra straps with these concealers.

- **No See 'Ems™.** With these double-sided tape strips, you won't have a gap from a missing button. They are packaged like a matchbook to fit anywhere.

- **Insoles.** Achy toes? Hurting heels? Keep a cushy insole on hand (check out www.footpetals.com).

- **Band-Aids** are good for protecting blisters and other boo-boos.

- **Stain remover.** I like Stain Eraser™, a biodegradable wipe made by ChemFree® or the Tide-to-go stain eraser pen.

- **Lint sheets.** The Pocket-Packs made by Scotch™ are so cute! They fit in your purse and work like a charm.

- **Invisi-Sole.** This is a non-toxic (so they say!) polymer similar to rubber that you paint on any problem area of your shoe. It creates a clear cushion that cuts down friction (www.invisi-sole.com).

- **Nail file, nail clippers, black marker, tissues.** And whatever else suits your needs.

If you don't feel like making your own kit, try the *She*mergency Survival Kit™ made by Ms. & Mrs. It contains a folding hair brush with mirror, hairspray, hair elastics, earring backs, hand lotion, nail clippers, emery board, clear nail polish, nail polish remover, mending kit, safety pin, double-sided tape, lint remover, shoe shine wipes, stain remover, static remover, breath freshener, lip balm, dental floss, pain reliever, deodorant wipes, tampon, adhesive bandages and facial tissues . . . all for $20! Visit www.msandmrs.com.

## Throw a Fashion Swap

You can do this at a women's group or with friends and family; it's a great way to freshen up your wardrobe, recycle and save money, all at the same time.

1. Decide on the date of your swap party and invite everyone you think has cool clothes. Invite at least two people of similar size and be sensitive to people of various shapes. Make it seasonal— it will force you and others to clean out your closets four times a year. Sample invitation:

   Hi, fellow fashion lovers! I've decided I need some new clothes, but I don't want to spend any money . . . so I have decided to throw a FASHION SWAP! Looking through my closet, I see all these great clothes that I'm a bit tired of or that I have trouble getting into (because I eat too much salad). I know some of you might love them, so come to my place on Saturday at 5:30 p.m. Before then, clean out your own closet and bring clothes and jewelry to swap. The more you bring, the more you get! Try to have all the items washed and pressed, just like you want to find your "new" clothes, brought by other people.

Please RSVP. Shelly.

2. Designate three "value spots" on a table or on the floor. Mark them as "Cheap," "Midprice" and "Expensive." Create different-colored tickets for each pile, about 20 for each. Leave a spot for people to write their names. (Multi-colored slips of construction paper work just as well as fancy tickets.)

3. Have at least two full-length mirrors so that the guests can see themselves. Put some cool music on for a festive mood. You can also have some finger foods or snacks.

4. When your guests arrive, tell them to put each item they brought in the value spot that they think suits it best. For each item they put down, give them a corresponding ticket. Ask them to write their names on each ticket they receive. (For every item they brought, they will get to pick an item from the same pile.)

5. Once all the items have been sorted, collect all the tickets and put them in a hat or box.

6. Shake up all the tickets and then draw one. The person whose name you draw gets to pick a clothing item from the corresponding pile.

7. When that person has made her selection, draw another name.

8. If one person chooses an item that somebody else really wants, play a game to decide who wins. Try Rock-Paper-Scissors or Charades.

9. If there are clothes left at the end of the swap, donate the rest to the charity of your choice.[7]

If a party is too much trouble, you can swap online at www.swap style.com, www.restylexchange.com or www.myfashionswap.com.

Whether you swap, keep, sell, donate or buy new, next time you put on an outfit, remember the three-point check. Ask yourself, *What are my clothes saying about me?* Remember: Your attire is a reflection of who you are.

# Nine

## Luxury Living for Less

sat on my backyard swing and gazed into a landscape of beautiful trees, knowing that this sanctuary would soon be only a memory. Leaves danced in the breeze accompanied by an orchestra of birds, but I was unable to move . . . not because I was physically paralyzed, but because my poor choices had bound me and limited my freedom.

What I did was irresponsible—I was selfish, anxious and spontaneous, and my family were the ones who suffered. If something looked good, I bought it. A new trend, I tried it. A good sale, I found it. I had no budget, and didn't care to make one.

I soon learned a bargain is not a bargain if it's not within a budget.

Why am I telling you all this? Because I hope you won't have to sell your home, like I did, because of poor choices, poor planning and a poor budget.

I learned the hard way that living above your means buys you instant gratification and long-term financial suffering. I was never taught how to save money. My dad's only words of financial advice were, "Don't borrow from strangers," and "If you don't have cash, don't buy it." When I finally took the Financial Peace University course by Dave Ramsey, I was more than ready to learn to manage my money! When I took the class, it was too late for me to fix our current situation but not too late to change the future of our finances.

Dave's humorous approach won me over, and now I'm on a tight leash. I value money, but financial resources are not a god. I want to handle money with wisdom, not with carelessness and selfishness.

Whether you have made the same mistakes I've made or have long lived wisely with money, you make daily decisions about how to prioritize your expenses . . . including those on personal care. Living a "rich" life doesn't necessarily mean spending a lot of money. You can surround yourself with beauty and can care for yourself in beautiful ways while still managing your finances wisely.

# OVERCOME OVERSPENDING

The first step to "living rich for less" is to correct any negative financial habits you have developed. If you are an overspender and want to make wiser money choices, try following these steps to correct your finances and live a simpler, yet beautiful, life.

## Admit You Spend Too Much

This is an absolute first step. As any alcoholic or drug addict knows, you cannot change what you do not acknowledge. Ask forgiveness from God and from your family. Seek out a program that can help you, such as the Financial Peace University course (www.daveramsey.com) or Crown Financial Ministries (www.crown.org), and consider a debt consolidation or counseling organization.

## Go on a "Debt-Fast"

No spending for 30 days, except for the absolute essentials (groceries, gas, utilities . . . and cut down on those, too!). Make it a game! For instance, see how many meals you can make out of what's already in your refrigerator, freezer and pantry. Walk or take public transportation to cut down on travel expenses. Play games or do puzzles with your kids instead of going to a movie or to the mall. Get creative. I bet you can come up with lots of ways to make your family's debt-fast fun.

Fasting from habitual spending will help you gain some perspective on how much you spend and on what. Think about it: If you buy a grande coffee at Starbucks every day, that's $60 a month . . . and that's just for drip! Why not spend $20 instead on two pounds of organic, fair-trade coffee and brew it at home every day?

## Cut Up Your Credit Cards

Yep, this is a tough one. Plastic surgery time, ladies! You can't charge on it if it's not there. Do yourself a favor and take the first step toward kicking debt out of your life for good. Shred it, burn it, let the dog chew on it, *whatever* . . . get rid of it!

## Fight the Impulse to Spend

Impulse spending will negatively impact your financial future, and it can be hard to fight the urge. Try one or all of these tricks when you get that "feeling"—the sweaty palms, the pounding heart and the knee-jerk reaction to reach for your purse. Take a breath. Tell yourself you can buy the item after you've thought about it for 30 days. Keep a little notepad in your purse and make an "I want to buy . . ." list. Write down all the things you're tempted to purchase, and then review the list after two weeks or a month. Chances are that, given a little time, you'll think to yourself, *Why did I think I needed that?* If you still want to buy the item, talk it over with an accountability partner, your spouse or a close girlfriend. If they agree that you can afford it and that the purchase is a wise use of your money, buy it with cash and let the guilt go.

## Recognize that Budgets (and Diets) Don't Work

You're probably thinking, *Is she kidding?* According to Sharon Durling, author of *A Girl and Her Money*, budgets and diets don't work, but lifestyle changes do. Outer constraints only make us grumpy; they don't help us change on the inside. Shannon suggests that you start the transformation by spending below your means, keeping a journal to pinpoint problems, and digging to get to the roots of the issue. As you're honest with yourself, you'll learn exactly where your money problems arise— maybe from envy, insecurity or fear. As you and God deal with these interior issues, you can begin to make practical choices to save money, such as turning the hot water heater and the air conditioner down a few degrees, switching off lights when you leave a room, and shutting off the water when you brush your teeth. (These are money- *and* eco-friendly tips!) This "save" rather than "spend" mentality will spill over into other areas of your life as well.[1]

Self-discipline, resourcefulness and self-awareness will help you discover a new lifestyle that brings financial peace.

## Make Some Money

If you need to pay off debt, check out www.womenforhire.com—you'll find résumé pointers, job listings and tips from women who have landed jobs. You can sign up to have listings sent to your inbox via www.mon ster.com and www.careerbuilder.com. There are quite a number of work-at-home opportunities, as well.

Also try digging around in your home, attic or garage for items to sell at a consignment store, on an auction site (such as www.ebay.com) or in a yard sale to pay off some of your debt.

## GREAT WAYS TO SAVE

Here are some amazing and fun ways to save, have fun and live in luxury for less!

## Everyday Savings

### *Secondhand Deals*

Shop in secondhand stores, consignment shops, vintage stores and flea markets. It's amazing what you can find at these fun little shops for unbelievably low prices! On www.thethriftshopper.com, you can find the locations of your local charity or church secondhand stores. Also check out discount department stores such as TJ Maxx, Marshalls and Target for good buys on household items, clothing, electronics and shoes. Another site to take a peak at: www.yardsalequeen.com.

### *eBay and Amazon.com*

These are both great places to shop online for used books, movies, music and other items. *Tip*: To avoid impulse spending on Amazon.com, opt out of "One-Click" purchasing and add items to your wish-list for at least seven days before you buy.

## Outlet Stores

Outlets are great places to find bargains on clothes and housewares. Check out children's clothing stores at the end of each season and there's a good chance you'll find shorts for $.99 or winter coats for $10.

## Trade with Others

If you have kids, start a clothes-trading circle with some of your girlfriends, or offer to buy their children's hand-me-downs at garage-sale prices. This is a great way to get quality clothes at a fraction of the retail price (or for nothing at all!). Brainstorm other ways to barter your time or resources for items or services you need.

## Carpool

Ride together to save gas and time. Check out www.dividetheride.com; this free site can help your group get organized—it even generates a schedule!

## Do Your Own Drycleaning

I know, I know . . . you can't really do your own drycleaning. But you can get clothes professionally cleaned less frequently if you purchase a steamer and "clean" them on your own. Lightly spritz your item with a fabric refresher (you can make your own using water, distilled vinegar and a few drops of your favorite essential oil) and then steam.

## Build Wealth

When shopping with cash, use only bills for purchases, and then save the change (a friend of mine once paid for a vacation this way). When using your debit card, round off your purchases at the dollar and put the difference in your savings account.

Let your bank help. Did you know that Bank of America has a "keep the change" program? They will match your savings at 100 percent for three months. My husband just received $250 from Regions Bank simply by signing up for a new business account. Check out your local bank for available deals.

If you have discipline (and *only* if you have the discipline) to pay off credit cards monthly, look for cards that give cash back. One card from American Express deposits 1 percent of your total purchases, plus a $50 bonus after your first purchase.

### Save on Gas

When you pump, keep the flow going slow; pumping too quickly wastes gas. Also, regular unleaded gas works just as well as the higher-priced fuels for fewer cents per gallon, according to the standards set by the Environmental Protection Agency. Do a little research online to find out if your area has a website that tracks prices; it may be worth your while to go out of your way for great savings.

### Pay Less at the Grocery Store

Check out www.groceryguide.com to track down the sales and best prices at your local supermarkets. Find unadvertised sales on www.fabu.com and www.retailmenot.com.

### Get a Scholarship

If you're eligible, a single mother can get up to $1,000 in scholarship money from www.raisethenation.org. If you're over 35, the Jeannette Rankin Foundation awards needs-based scholarships from www.rankin foundation.org. Others to look into are www.militaryscholar.org if you or a family member is in the military.

### Movie Night In

Netflix members receive unlimited video rentals for a monthly subscription price. Blockbuster also offers unlimited rentals, both through the mail and in stores.

### Track Down the Deals

Check out www.shefinds.com, a funny, girl-friendly site that advises you on seasonal deals and other good online buys.

## Travel in Style

### Family Vacation Tips

Check out John Tesh's website, www.tesh.com, for great travel tips, like these ideas for sticking to your travel budget while on vacation:

- If you'd like discounts at theme parks, check out eBay and do a search for "theme park tickets." You'll find all kinds of two-for-one deals, family packs, and discounts for theme parks everywhere.

- If you plan to hit a few national parks, like Yosemite, Yellowstone, and the Grand Canyon, those 3 entry fees alone will cost you $60 . . . get a Parks Pass at NationalParks.org. For $50, your whole family can get into *any* national park in the U.S. free for a whole year!

- If you're going to a major city, like New York, Chicago, or Hollywood, try CityPass.com. A pass can save you up to 50 percent when you visit several tourist attractions in the area.

- And one final trick for saving money on your next "vay-kay." When you're looking for souvenirs, avoid the gift shops and hit the local Costco or Wal-Mart. According to travel expert Pauline Frommer, superstores carry the same T-shirts and postcards minus the tourist price-hikes.[2]

### Luggage

Look for quality luggage at a good price at discount stores such as TJ Maxx, Marshalls and Tuesday Morning. Garage and estate sales are other good options for finding high-quality luggage. If you're ever in Scotsboro, Alabama, check out the Unclaimed Baggage Center; you can get great deals on luggage and other items that have been left behind at airports (visit www.unclaimedbaggage.com for more info).

### Cruises

A cruise may not be as far out of reach as you may think. Check out www.cruisedeals.com.

### Timeshare Tours

Sure it's a little awkward to reject the sales offer after you've stayed at the property and taken the tour, but hey—your financial future is at stake. So take the tour and enjoy the weekend. But *just say no!* If you're not good at saying no, skip this option.

### Share the Cost

Share a vacation with several girlfriends and split the cost of a nice hotel. My friend Lisa and her two sisters stayed at the Hyatt Regency in Wichita, Kansas—right on the Arkansas River—for $60 from Priceline.com. The regular room rate is about $210, but it cost each only $20 for the most beautiful hotel in town. Not bad, huh?

### Check for Last-Minute Deals

This is a fantastic way to travel inexpensively. Travel websites such as www.priceline.com, www.travelocity.com, www.sidestep.com, www.farecast.com and www.expedia.com are good sources for last-minute vacation packages, hotel rooms, flights and rental cars.

### Travel in the Off-Season

This is particularly helpful if you like to hang out at the beach or at a ski resort. Prices drop dramatically just a few days after the "end" of the season. Who says you can't hit the beach in the fall or ski in April? Some slopes are even open until the Fourth of July.

### Explore Your Own Backyard

What can you see in your own city for less? In many areas, you can visit museums or historical sites for free or for very little money. How about taking in a high school or college sporting event at a fraction of the cost of a pro game? Take your family to a park or conservation area; play, relax and take in God's beautiful creation without spending a penny. And don't forget the public library . . . it's not just a great bargain for books, music and movie lovers: Many public libraries also offer seminars, family fun days (or nights), story time for kids and even movie nights—all at no cost to you.

*Travel from Your Armchair*

Watch the Travel Channel or read about your ideal vacation spot. I have been to Spain, Austria, France, Italy, and many other exotic locales by watching the Travel Channel or PBS specials. Public libraries often carry lots of travel magazines, so you can take a (mental) vacation without spending a dime. Keep brochures or travel articles about places you'd like to visit in a "someday" file for when you're financially able to travel.

*And a few more travel tips . . .*

1. Dress well and up your odds of a flight upgrade (fees are lower if there are empty seats on the plane). First class, baby!

2. Check into becoming a travel agent. My friend does this on the side; she makes money and gets to travel *cheap*.

3. Stay at a cheaper hotel and book a spa treatment at a nearby more expensive resort.

## Dine on a Dime

- Eat at a nice restaurant for lunch instead of dinner. It's usually cheaper, and the portion sizes tend to be smaller, which is great for your outer beauty.

- Use the discounts offered in your local *Entertainment*® *Book*.

- When traveling, ask the locals where they eat. You'll be more likely to find lesser-known (but just as delicious) restaurants and cafés. Avoid tourist-trap restaurants.

- Order appetizers instead of main dishes, share a meal with your spouse or friend, and opt for water as a beverage.

- Look for dining coupons in your local paper and in your junk mail.

- Find out when during the week your local restaurants have specials.

- Seek out grand openings.

- Join www.idine.com—restaurants that participate give you 20 percent off your bill. The Rewards Network™ retains the first $49 you earn; after that, it's all yours. Members have earned a few hundred to a few thousand dollars.

- Many restaurants have a kids-eat-free night or a buy-one-get-one-free special one evening a week.

- Take half of your dinner home for the next day's lunch. Restaurant portion sizes are outrageous these days, and taking half home cuts the calories in half and stretches the money twice as far. Some dishes, such as pasta, taste even better the second time around.

- Order a kid's meal for yourself; I do when I go out. Servers are usually accommodating, but if you don't ask, you'll never know!

## Household Items and Services

One hot, sunny, melting Florida day, I went to visit some garage sales with my husband (I usually go with Mom). I was seven-months pregnant, and I was hungry (imagine how sweet and compliant I was!).

Well, I saw this dining set and I just *had* to have it: antique cherry wood and oh-so beautiful. The price was $400. I looked at my husband with sad, puppy-dog eyes. He said a flat, "No."

That answer did not sit with me too well; I wanted it and I wanted it *now*. I pouted all the way back to the car and gave him my "attack" puppy-dog eyes. I picked up the newspaper in the car and saw an ad for a brand-name dining set with a china cabinet and buffet for $1,400. I asked if we could go to the furniture store and look at it, expecting Angelo to repeat his earlier answer. To my surprise, he said yes.

It was love at first sight: blond wood, beautiful beveled glass with mirrors in the cabinet, plenty of storage at the base. I looked at my husband and begged, "*Pleeeeeeeease!* I'll do anything . . ."

We got the price down to $1,100 and walked away with a beautiful set that we still love more than 10 years later.

The moral of this story is: *Don't settle* (and, sometimes your husband is right). Diligently search for the best quality merchandise for your money. Start your hunt at garage sales in high-end neighborhoods, on www.craigslist.com, at estate sales and Goodwill stores. Ask your friends if they know anyone selling furniture (or whatever you're looking for). For household items and furnishings, check stores like Ikea, Tuesday Morning, American Signature (there are great bargains near the back of the store), Target and other discount stores. Look for bigger sale discounts when seasons change (e.g., Christmas in January and summer items in August). Shop end-of-season clearance sales, especially at discount stores or outlet malls.

Barter and trade for items and services. If you can cut hair and your friend cleans houses, trade. Can you tutor a child in reading or math, mend clothes, groom dogs or teach piano lessons? Get creative, ask around, and before long you'll be bartering for all you're worth.

## Recreation

Use recreation discounts in your local *Entertainment Book* for the theatre, opera, movies, bowling . . . you name it. Go with friends or family to get a group discount for some recreational activities, such as miniature golf.

Gather at the home of a friend who has a pool or ping-pong table, or to watch a sporting event together. Each family can bring snack foods to make a great party for little expense.

## *Trés Chic* Eco-Friendly and Creative Giving

- Make your own signature gifts for friends; Jackie Kennedy did. Does everyone rave about your homemade chocolate-chip cookies or blueberry muffins? Put them in pretty boxes or old tins and give them as gifts. Are you an amateur photographer? Offer to take your friend's kid's picture for her birthday. Do you make jewelry or candles? Do you sew? The possibilities are endless.

- Give a planting/seed greeting card set. The recipient gets to plant the seed or planting and watch it grow.

- Find inexpensive items and create beautiful gifts. For instance, use a mason jar and layer it with bath salts, flower petals and herbs, then top with a ribbon. Or burn a special CD of songs for friends and family. Or take empty colored bottles of varying sizes, fill with water and baby's breath, and place on a tray for a beautiful mixed-glass centerpiece for lunch with friends or a shower. Or make your own soaps or aromatherapy spray bottles to give as gifts.

- Buy in bulk when gift or craft items go on sale.

- Be a deal hunter. Shop the endcaps and the backs of stores. I got a beautiful etched-glass bathroom vanity mirror at Target for $7 (it was originally $40) and found a designer shirt at Macy's for $30, marked down from $275. My shopping buddy LeAnn got a $599 jacket for $40 and her $799 Inaugural ball gown for $120 after coupons on the day-after-Christmas sale. At JC Penney, she got a $500 men's suit for $18—I saw the price tag and the receipt . . . what a fantastic deal! And what a great gift for a husband, father or friend.

## Pamper Your Inner Princess [3]

- Get hair styled, massages and manicures/pedicures at local beauty/massage schools. You will feel pampered at a fraction of the cost. In addition, some health insurances now honor 25 percent off a massage; find out if your insurance will, too.

- Go to Brookstone and try out one of their massage chairs for free. I do it when I go to the mall, and it feels great (it also gives you a second wind for more bargain shopping).

- Go for a polish change instead of a full pedicure at a posh salon.

- Want a beautiful wall hanging? Buy a large coffee table art book (lots of these go on sale at local bookstores) or a beautiful calendar with photos, then rip out the pages and buy some frames at Michaels (use their 50-percent-off coupon from the newspaper) or any discount store. Even simple black or white frames look lovely.

- Get a free makeover at the beauty counter in the mall.

- Quench your thirst in luxury. I bought a Sigg™ reusable water bottle (check out your local health food store) and it is so beautiful. I love the fact that I am helping the environment and saving about $1,000 a year by filling it myself.

- Get a fashionable bag for a bargain-basement price at www.bag haus.com.

- For stylish (and affordable!) sunglasses, check out www.bleu dame.com.

- Plant a moon garden. Fill planters with night-blooming jasmine, tuberose, honeysuckle, morning glory and night phlox. Place some garden candles around and enjoy relaxing in your evening paradise.

- Travel like a princess. Pack a mini-lunch in a beautiful case with royal snacks, such as cucumber sandwiches, pimento-and-olive sandwiches and grapes, and a thermos of organic tea. Don't forget a monogrammed hankie instead of a paper napkin!

- Make a lavender sachet with sprigs and buds, place in a swatch of vintage fabric and tie it at the top with ribbon. Place under your pillow in the morning when you make the bed. When you're ready to turn in, flip the pillow over and get a good night's fragrant sleep. Store the sachet in a bedside drawer or leave it on your nightstand.

- If you have an office, take a princess break. Open your desk drawer to a mini-oasis—peppermint lotion/foot spray, massage ball, aromatherapy inhaler (lavender for stress, citrus for energizing), an herbal tea bag and a tea cup—and take a break. Listen to some relaxing music on your iPod and enjoy.

## Splurges and Indulgences

If you've put a little "funny" money aside, here's what to splurge on:

### Have a Solo Sleepover

Book a night just for you at a bed and breakfast. *Hint*: You can get the best rate during the week. Take a nap, read, soak in a bubble bath, paint your toenails or watch chick flicks. Enjoy the solitude and use it as a time of pampering and refreshment. The next morning, start your day right with the fabulous breakfast that's included in your rate.

### Get a Good Haircut, Facial or Massage

Ask for gift cards to your favorite salon for your birthday, Christmas or Mother's Day. Then you won't feel guilty when you indulge yourself at the spa. For a massage, consider visiting your local massage school; instead of paying $75 or more, you'll pay about $25 for the same service. Find one near you at www.amtamassage.org.

### See a Movie at the Cinema

Making this a habit can wreck your budget, but it's fun as an occasional splurge—movies just aren't the same on your home TV screen! Make it a date with hubby, take the kids or go it alone.

### Buy a New Outfit

If you ask yourself the four *F*s before taking out your cash—Does it *fit*? Is it *functional*? Is it *flattering*? Is it *fabulous*?—and plan in advance to make a purchase, don't worry (too much) about the price tag. If the answer to each question is a resounding "Yes!" then you go, girl!

### Give It Away

Give the "blow money," as Dave Ramsey calls it, to someone in need. Do you know a single mom who could really use a movie date with her kids? Why not give a gift to the American Cancer Society or American Heart Association in honor of a loved one? People all over the world, including right where you live, are sick, hurting and desperate; use some of your available money to reach out to them. I guarantee, you'll never miss that massage or new outfit.

## A RICH LIFE

You can enjoy a beautiful life and not go into debt. I hope you don't have to repeat my experience of serious debt to learn your financial lesson. Know that life is so much more than money, more than stuff, more than all the external trappings of this world we live in. Jesus made a point of this in the Sermon on the Mount:

> *Do not store up for yourselves treasures on earth, where moth and rust destroy, and where thieves break in and steal. But store up for yourselves treasures in heaven, where moth and rust do not destroy, and where thieves do not break in and steal. For where your treasure is, there your heart will be also* (Matt. 6:19-21).

We learn from our Lord in these passages that changing our financial lives really begins with changing our focus—from our little kingdoms to His eternal kingdom. Trust our Father when He says that if you live in the pursuit of His righteousness, your life will be rich and beautiful indeed.

# Ten

# Scents and Sensibilities

oco Chanel once said, "No elegance is possible without perfume." Some of my fondest memories of fragrance are of my dad and the smell of Old Spice. Before he walked out the door to go to work, he'd give me a quick kiss, leaving behind a trail of the scent on my cheek.

My grandmother (Dad's mother) was also a fan of fragrance; her favorites were Elizabeth Taylor's perfumes. Grandmother, too, left a scent in her wake; but she hugged me so tight that I thought I would burst (and I loved it).

My mom was devoted to Estée Lauder White Linen, but now she has branched out. She has quite a fragrance collection (I buy natural perfumes for her, and she's starting to like them).

Funny how some of us stick with a certain scent forever and some of us change our fragrance as often as we switch outfits.

I used to wonder why I liked certain fragrances, while others gave me a headache or made me nauseous. Finally, more than a decade ago, I realized that I am extremely sensitive to chemicals in perfumes and in household products. After researching perfumes and their scented counterparts (including lotions and powders), I was surprised at what I discovered . . . and at the same time, I was relieved.

Before I tell you about my findings, let's find what type of scent you like.

## FRAGRANCE CATEGORIES

Most fragrances, whether in perfumes and colognes, oils or household products, fall into a few basic categories. Which are your favorites?

*Floral*: jasmine, gardenia, rose, lavender, ylang-ylang
*Citrus*: lemon, grapefruit, orange, lime, tangerine
*Musk*: patchouli, ambergris, musk
*Herbal*: rosemary, thyme, sage
*Green*: leaves, grass
*Woodsy*: oak, cedar, sandalwood

The sweet, white flower of ylang-ylang can be found growing in the Comoros Islands, off the coast of East Africa. Vanilla beans—try Madagascar. Jasmine and sandalwood originate from India. Mandarin comes from Sicily and lime oil from Mexico.

Beautiful rose scents often come from Turkey, Morocco or Bulgaria. There are distinct differences between various rose aromas, and some are more expensive than others. Roses are picked in the early hours to obtain the greatest essence, and once picked, weighed and bagged, the petals must be processed within 12 hours. It takes two tons of petals to produce one pound of Bulgarian rose oil.[1]

> *Did you know . . . ?*
>
> ❧ Arabs discovered how to distill petals and produce rose water, which they used in perfume and to scent food.

## FRAGRANCE NOTES

A specific characteristic of one of these categories is called a *note*. Most fragrances consist of three levels of notes:

**Top (head) notes** last for about half an hour. Head notes reach our sense of smell first, forming the scent's initial impression and then dissipating. Many head notes are familiar from cooking: herbs and spices such as coriander, spearmint, black pepper, cardamom, juniper, basil and tarragon; and citruses such as lime, bitter orange, blood orange, tangerine and pink grapefruit.

**Middle (heart) notes** last about two hours. These generally consist of the florals—geranium, rose, jasmine, orange flower, tuberose, violet leaf and ylang-ylang. Heady, dramatic, intense and sometimes sickly sweet, heart notes give body to blends, impart warmth and fullness and bring out the best in the other notes.

**Bottom (base) notes** last for several hours and as long as a few days. Intense and profound, base notes are often thick and syrupy, and most are derived from bark (sandalwood), roots (angelica), resins (labdanum), lichens (oak moss), saps (benzoin, peru balsam) and grasses (patchouli, vetiver).

## FRAGRANCE TYPES

The best places on the body to apply your perfume are at your pulse points. Or you can spray *once* and walk through it. When you apply fragrance, be sure to remove jewelry first, as it can lose its luster from exposure to perfumes, especially pearls.

Be aware of people around you who might have fragrance allergies or sensitivities—meaning, don't bathe in your fragrance before you leave home! People should notice *you* first, not your perfume.

Personal fragrances are found in a variety of forms for use on the body:

*Perfumes*: highest ratio of pure fragrance oil to alcohol
*Colognes*: more diluted with alcohol, cost less than perfume
*Body splashes or sprays*: lowest concentration of fragrance or
   essential oils

*Scented lotions*: lotions mixed with perfumes

*Solid perfumes*: essential oils mixed with beeswax, jojoba oil or other oils

You can make your own solid perfume, using this recipe:

1 tbsp. beeswax
1 tbsp. almond oil or jojoba oil
8 to 15 drops essential oil* of your choice
1 container (small sealable case made of glass, ceramic, stone or sterling silver)

*Pour about an inch of water in a small saucepan, then put a small glass jar or Pyrex bowl in the water. Measure out the beeswax and almond/jojoba oil into the jar/bowl and then bring the water around it to a boil. The wax will melt gradually. When it is 100-percent liquid, remove from heat and stir in remaining ingredients with a straw. (The wax will start to solidify on whatever you stir with; a straw has little surface area, so you lose less of the end product. It's also disposable, so you don't have to clean it off.) When everything is thoroughly mixed, pour the liquid wax immediately into your final container. In about 30 minutes, it will be cooled, solid and ready to use. Keep sealed to store.*

**BBG TIP**

I see a lot of companies out there advertising "natural" cosmetics and fragrances, but when you check the ingredients, it's just not true. Most fragrances are 95-percent synthetic chemicals, and few have been tested for their safety.

## BEHIND THE NOTES

Stacy Malkan, author of *Not Just a Pretty Face: The Ugly Side of the Beauty Industry*, explains best why I became so irritated with fragrances. Much of the irritation I experienced—and perhaps you have as well—comes from toxins and chemicals included in many fragrant products. Some hidden hazards that may be lurking within synthetic/chemical fragrances include:

- **Allergens:** Fragrances are among the top-five known allergens, and can both cause asthma and trigger asthma attacks.

- **Phthalates:** We learned about these in chapter 4. Manufacturers usually won't name these in their ingredient lists.

* Bergamot, patchouli, civet, galbanum and asafetida can pose problems for more sensitive cosmetic users. With that in mind, use one oil at a time or no more than three to avoid an allergic response.

● **Sensitizers:** One in every 50 people may suffer immune system damage from fragrance and become sensitized. Once sensitized to an ingredient, a person can remain so for a lifetime, enduring chronic allergic reactions.[2]

As far back as 1986, Malkan reports, the U.S. National Academy of Sciences identified fragrance ingredients as one of six categories of neurotoxins (toxic to the brain) that should be thoroughly investigated for their impact on human health.[3]

Now, I know some of you are saying, "I'm not giving up my perfume even if it gives me a headache." I'm not asking you to. I just want you to know what you are putting on your skin and how it may affect your health.

Perfumer Mandy Aftel, author of *Essence and Alchemy*, has been featured on CNN and in *Vogue, Vanity Fair, In Style, TIME* and many other publications. She offers great information on the difference between natural and synthetic perfumes. Aftel defines "natural" perfume as having essential oils, "absolutes," "concrete," $CO_2$ extracts and resins as ingredients.

I had a chance to speak with Mandy, who is also the owner of Aftelier perfumes (one of my favorites from her line is Pink Lotus, originally created for Madonna). "My approach to creating artisan natural perfumes is based in the quality and integrity of the ingredients," she explains. "Unlike most commercial perfumes, for each of my hand-crafted liquid and solid perfumes, I choose from among more than five hundred of the finest natural essences found anywhere in the world, using organic or wild-crafted oils whenever possible."[4] She continues:

Natural perfume can be considered art when constructed correctly, and always made by hand. Discovering the art of natural perfumery is like crossing the threshold of a beautiful old house and finding it utterly intact and splendidly furnished—but deserted, as if it had been suddenly abandoned. It took centuries to discover ways of extracting scent from aromatic materials. Yet just as a full palette of natural essences became available, commercial perfumers began to set them aside in favor of synthetic ingredients, which are cheaper, sturdier and more uniform in quality. Unfortunately, they have none of the richness or complexity of the natural ingredients, and they result in "linear" fragrances that strike the senses bluntly, all at once.[5]

Today, almost every perfume is created from synthetic essences. Although synthetics approximate the odors of natural ingredients, they have none of the complexity, mystery or emotional depth.

## SURROUND YOURSELF WITH BEAUTY

When I talk about surrounding yourself with beauty, I don't mean with a bunch of synthetic junk like cheap candles and plug-in devices that emit more chemicals. We already live in a chemical soup from our environment and our own homes (as we explored in chapter 6), so why would we add more fuel to the fire?

I had the pleasure of interviewing Athena Thompson, a certified building biologist and author of *Homes that Heal (and Those that Don't)*. I asked her about candles and the usage of essential oils. Here's what she had to say:

> Anytime you use combustible products, you will have combustible by-products. I do have beeswax candles—unscented. I don't use anything with synthetic fragrance. Many candles advertised as "aromatherapy candles" are not using organic essential oils, so they are using essential oils that have been distilled using chemicals. If you want candles for ambiance, I suggest unscented. If you want a background aroma, ask yourself why: Is it to mask a bad smell, is it because you don't open your windows and let fresh air and oxygen in, or do you just like your home to smell fragranced?
>
> If you want some aroma, then organic essential oils are the best way to go . . . but don't overdo it. I never heat essential oils.

I use a small battery-powered fan dispenser—great for travel and staying in hotels. With essential oils you have to make sure you know what you are doing, as you will breathe the essential oils into your lungs, sinuses, etc. Some people react even to organic essential oils. It's simpler if you use single essential oils, i.e. lavender, than some of these popular oil "blends."

But there is no replacement for good, oxygenated, fresh air![6]

Why not open the windows? Unless you live by a highway, opening the windows is the best way to let bad air out and good air in. And allowing sunlight into your home and supplementing with full-spectrum lighting in darker rooms, Thompson says, "is equivalent to giving your home a tonic. Plus, the UV-C ray, which is mostly filtered out by the Earth's ozone layer, is germicidal, killing bacteria, viruses, and other infectious agents."[7]

So let the sunshine in!

> Many common indoor plants can reduce certain toxic chemicals in the air. Place plants at 100-foot intervals to remove pollutants from in your home.
>
> **BBG TIP**

While the sun is shining through the windows, let the rays add life to beautiful, air-purifying plants. Did you know that plants remove toxins? For instance, a Boston fern helps remove air pollutants, especially formaldehyde, and adds humidity to an indoor environment. The *ficus alii* is a large plant that also helps purify the air and remove chemical vapors (please check the Resource section at the end of this book for a list of air-cleaning plants).

I do enjoy subtle fragrance around the house, but I changed from synthetic paraffin candles to aromatherapy soy or beeswax candles. I use distilled diffusers from Young Living Essential Oils (youngliving.us) and Mountain Rose Herbs (www.mountainroseherbs.com).

## THIRTY DAYS OF ELEGANCE

Surrounding your life with beauty is not just about fragrance; you can create and discover the essence of elegance in everyday life. The definition of "elegance" is "tastefully luxurious." I invite you to create little pockets of pleasure for one month. Whether you are helping a friend out or indulging in a luxurious bath, it's the little things in life that make a difference in your attitude and outlook. Nothing is more "fragrant" than a positive, giving approach to life.

**Day 1:** Write a note to someone you know in an assisted-living center.

**Day 2:** Begin a "grateful journal" and write one thing you are thankful for each day (keep it at your bedside). When you're feeling down, read it!

**Day 3:** Collect some flowers and place them in your kitchen.

**Day 4:** Drink your coffee or tea from an antique cup and saucer.

**Day 5:** Learn one French or Italian word for the next 30 days.

**Day 6:** Read a novel by Jane Austen or another classic author.

**Day 7:** Watch *Breakfast at Tiffany's* or *Gigi*.

**Day 8:** Use a beaded or silver cup to hold Q-tips or cotton balls.

**Day 9:** Donate books or magazines to your local women's resource center or nursing home.

**Day 10:** Read some poetry.

**Day 11:** Write a poem or a song (I used to do this in high school and recently started again).

**Day 12:** Practice standing up straight; you'll appear taller and more confident.

**Day 13:** Listen to classical music or an opera. Maybe do a bit of research about the person who wrote the piece.

**Day 14:** Take out the good china, light some candles and eat in the dining room.

**Day 15:** Tame your tongue—no gossiping (we should do this every day, of course!).

**Day 16:** Buy someone a gift for no reason, or make something for a friend or relative.

**Day 17:** Visit your local garden club. Take a book to read, surrounded by the beauty God created. We have Leu Gardens here in Florida; I have a membership and love going there.

**Day 18:** Read a biography about someone who inspires you.

**Day 19:** Go to a tea room with a friend, mother, sister or daughter.

**Day 20:** Lose track of time at an art or history museum.

**Day 21:** Frame a Scripture verse or a quote that captivates you.

**Day 22:** Wear your expensive perfume today.

**Day 23:** Go to a park and sketch some nature (you don't have to be a great artist).

**Day 24:** Book a massage at a salon (or at a massage school for half the price).

**Day 25:** Wear a cashmere cardigan or scarf. Can't afford one? Pashmere is a soft, luxurious alternative; I bought a pashmina for $5.

**Day 26:** Watch the sunset or sunrise.

**Day 27:** Name your house. Why should the Biltmore have a name but not your place? Okay, it has 500 rooms where some of us have only 5. . . but name your castle anyway; it is your history. (How does Ballestero Cottage sound?)

**Day 28:** Drink your water from a goblet or enjoy a smoothie in a crystal glass.

**Day 29:** Draw a bath with essential oils, then soak to the sounds of soothing music and the glow of candlelight.

**Day 30:** Wear your pearls!

I know that, in the real world, it is hard to do even the simplest of these elegance exercises—much less make the switch to natural fragrance products. Yet if you do only one thing to create natural beauty and elegance around you, it *will* make a difference. You will reap the benefits, and so will your environment and those around you. Enjoy life as much as you can; God has filled it with beauty just for us, and given us family and friends to share our greatest achievements or grievous moments. He is the Creator of the first majestic landscape, as well as our lives, futures and eternal paradise. He is the greatest inventor of all time, and He has created a masterpiece—a fragrant, beautiful world—for us to live in and enjoy. Take the time to smell the roses; your heavenly Father made them just for you!

# Eleven

# Alleviate Stinkin' Thinkin'

Have you ever stopped to think about what you're thinking about? That might sound strange, but it's key to living the beautiful life God has planned for you. Inner beauty starts in your mind: Thoughts create feelings and attitudes; feelings and attitudes create actions; actions create habits; and habits create your character, which translates into who you are. To change the way you look, feel or act, you have to start at the same place: your thoughts.

## THE WHEELS IN THE MIND GO ROUND AND ROUND

To understand your attitudes about beauty, self-image and God, you have to define what thoughts are reflected by those attitudes. If thinking creates attitudes, then we have to change our thinking to reflect God's thoughts about beauty.

A good place to start when trying to change our thought patterns is to look at where our thoughts originate. Each of us defines beauty in our own way, but that definition is often formed by outside influences. Our earliest images of beauty are often of the women in our family—sisters, mother, grandmothers and aunts. In his book *Self-Talk: Key to Personal Growth*, Dr. David

Stoop explains that dysfunctional thought patterns begin in childhood, and that anyone who wants to change these patterns must work at understanding their family's influence: "Breaking free from their distorted self-talk required them to better understand their family of origin and its influence in their lives."[1] Take a step back in time and ask yourself these questions:

- Belief about myself: *What do I like or not like about myself?*

- Belief about others: *As a child, what do I remember thinking about adults? About teachers? About my friends' parents?*

- Belief about the world: *When I think about the future, what do I see? When I think about the past, what do I avoid?*

- Belief about God: *What is the hardest thing for me to experience in my relationship with God today?*

- Other beliefs: *How did we handle family conflicts? Who talked most in my family? Who didn't talk?*[2]

Think about how these early experiences influence your perception of yourself, others and the world today. I can't tell you how important it is to get a hold of our belief systems. Some of our beliefs are rational (based in reality) and help us cope with life's events, while some are irrational (not based in reality) and distort our ability to cope with life's ups and downs.

For years, I had irrational beliefs about men. I remember making a vow never again to get burned by a man—I was 21 years old, and so in love with my ex-boyfriend, Vin, who had broken up with me. To deal with my heartache, I smoked some weed and got a tattoo. (I know—I can't believe it either.) The tattoo is a heart in flames, representing that "I'll never get burned again." I swore that Vin would never see it.

Well, he did . . . and I got burned again. (That's what happens when you don't follow the will of God.) And I would have kept getting burned had I not closed the door on my past and on my irrational beliefs and behaviors.

"Distortions in your current perception of yourself are based on experiences accumulated over your lifetime in relationships with people you considered important or powerful."[3] The mind is like a computer system, and try as you might to act against its programming, your feelings and actions—however foolish and damaging—are controlled by its powerful software (that is, your beliefs), encoded by your early family experiences.

Our self-perceptions, whether wrong or right, began with our earliest relationships. Then, as we grew and were exposed to more and more images—on television, movies and magazine covers—more outside ideas about beauty were layered atop our existing perceptions, usually resulting in more negative self-talk. Unfortunately, in our sex-obsessed culture, most of our beliefs about beauty are unrealistic at best and unhealthy at worst. We know from

> Beauty is being in harmony with what you are.
>
> —Peter Nivio Zarlenga, *The Orator*

chapter 1 that computer-generated, airbrushed actresses and models don't look in real life like their pictures, so how can "normal" women like us possibly expect to?

Even if you're beautiful on the outside, your toxic insides might be obstructing the view because, ultimately, how we think about beauty and what we think about ourselves translates on the outside. Harsh, negative or critical thoughts never fit into God's definition of true beauty.

To make matters even worse, we internalize the "perfect" images we see and twist them into more than just pretty pictures. Before we realize it, achieving that kind of "perfection" has become our all-consuming quest. So, as we trudge out of the grocery store pushing a cart after seeing the waifs on the checkout line magazine racks, we feel discontent, discouraged and depressed. We start to feel inadequate and guilty, and then the mind games begin: We vow not to eat the junk we just liberated from the grocery store. *Why do I eat so much? Why don't I look like that? I hate the way I look.* On and on we go, tearing ourselves down and comparing ourselves with fiction. Or we go to the opposite extreme: *I'll never look like that, so why bother?* And we go home and eat all the junk we just bought. Both responses are destructive, and both are based on an unrealistic attitude derived from wrong thinking.

## Who Do We Listen To?

Wrong thinking always leads to wrong attitudes that negatively affect how we see ourselves. Negative thoughts from the past, along with today's unrelenting onslaught of media images, could keep us trapped in a bad self-image for a long time. Instead, God wants us to see ourselves through His eyes. The mind is a powerful thing, but by reading God's Word, we can begin to replace destructive thoughts, which lead to destructive behaviors, with His view of beauty, a view He wants to impart to all His children. But we have to make a choice about who (or what) we're going to listen to. Let's face it: Those movies and magazines aren't going anywhere—it's going to take a conscious effort to choose to listen to God's voice instead. Let the Father guide you through the past to sail into the promises of the Holy Scriptures.

> The wind will carry me,
> above my wildest dreams.
> Those storms and waves may
> follow me, but my spirit sails free.
> —Angelo Ballestero, "The Wind Will Carry Me"

## Understand the Power of the Mind

We've seen how powerful the mind is in controlling, even subconsciously, our attitudes, actions and habits. Replacing those thoughts takes effort and time, but our God-given minds *are* capable of learning to think on the right things. We must always remember that our behaviors and habits trace back to our thoughts.

If we are to change our perceptions, we have to change our minds. A transformed mind has the power to change our attitudes, behaviors and habits, so that we can reflect God's view of beauty, not a false view derived from stinkin' thinkin'.

> Do not conform any longer to the pattern of this world, but be transformed by the renewing of your mind. Then you will be able to test and approve what God's will is—his good, pleasing and perfect will (Rom. 12:2, *NIV*).

It sounds good to say that we need to listen to God's Word and think on the good things (which will help us think differently about ourselves), but it's not an easy change to make. After all, that old stinkin' thinkin' is buried deep inside. We have to be willing to really understand how we see ourselves now. And we have to really believe that God's view of beauty is the truth.

> *For as*
> *he thinks in*
> *his heart, so is he.*
> (Prov. 23:7, AMP).

## Why Be a Knockoff?

As we discussed in chapter 1, God's definition of beauty is that He created each of us to be a unique reflection of His own character. Each of us is gifted and beautiful in different ways; God planted a specific purpose into each of us before we were born. Instead of living freely in this truth, we are tempted to compare ourselves to those around us, feeding the comparisons with negative thoughts from our past.

We've already established that trying to become the Hollywood images we are constantly spoon-fed is not only unhealthy, it's impossible. But why would we ever want to be a knockoff of someone else in the first place? God made each of us unique for a reason. If God's idea of "perfection" was blonde and pencil-thin, that's how we would all look. Stop and think about that for a second. When we're caught in the comparison trap, the last thing we want is someone to remind us that God loves diversity and that He made us exactly the way He intended. But clichéd or not, that statement is full of truth—and freedom.

I have loved art since I was five years old. As I've grown older, my love of art has intensified as I've realized how art parallels life in many ways—not the least in its application to our definition of beauty. No one appreciates "cookie-cutter" art. Each piece's individuality is what makes it beautiful—just like us. True art isn't "cloneable"; people pay millions for a one-of-a-kind original, but knockoffs or reprints are virtually worthless. The *Venus de Milo* is a good example: The sculpture is missing arms, but it's still a stunning, priceless masterpiece. Michelangelo, *Venus de Milo's* creator, dedicated his life to the study of beauty. When he approached sculpting, he did not see the block of marble; he saw the beauty that was waiting inside. The idea of bringing inward beauty out consumed him; he expressed it through art, poetry, sculpting, architecture, painting, and everything else that he did.

We can easily understand this notion of beauty when it comes to art. But when it comes to the artistry that our master Creator put into us, we don't get it. We still compare ourselves to Barbie. Everything in our society screams at us that we aren't normal unless we look like the tabloid queens. Why are we so ready to believe this lie? The truth about us, as with art, is that what makes us unique is what makes us beautiful.

So how can we reprogram our minds to appreciate our uniquely beautiful qualities? Dr. Neil Anderson, in his book *Overcoming Negative Self-Image*, puts it this way: "The more you reaffirm who you are in Christ, the more your behavior will reflect your true identity."[4] Pastor Joel Osteen has this to say about the importance of affirming ourselves, just the way we are, right now:

> We talk more to ourselves than we do to anyone else. And sometimes we've been doing it for so long, that it is like a record that plays over and over. This can either be good or bad. It depends on how we are talking to ourselves. What do you meditate on? Positive thoughts? Empowering thoughts? Affirming thoughts? Or do you go around like a lot of people thinking negative, defeated thoughts . . . "I'm unattractive." "I'm not talented." "I've made a lot of mistakes." "I'm sure God is not pleased with me." This negative self-talk is what keeps people from rising higher.[5]

The psalmist's plea should be ours, too: "May the words of my mouth and the meditations of my heart be acceptable in your sight, O LORD, my Rock and my Redeemer" (Ps. 19:14).

## REPROGRAM YOUR STINKIN' THINKIN'

We want to have the right perspective on beauty. We want to have the right attitude about who we are in God. We want to have a healthy self-image.

We know the Bible tells us that the key is to keep our thoughts on God and reaffirm who we are in Christ. All this is true, but how do we do it?

## Replace Your Thoughts

As we've seen, the mind is powerful. But you *can* control your mind and change how it affects the way you think about yourself. The following Scripture is a great place to start: "We demolish arguments and every pretension that sets itself up against the knowledge of God, and we take captive every thought to make it obedient to Christ" (2 Cor. 10:5). This is the foundation for changing our thinking: taking our thoughts captive. When you have a wrong or negative thought about yourself, stop and catch that thought before it goes any further.

But as we know, if we empty out a space, something else must take its place. So when you've stopped a destructive thought, you can't just leave a vacuum; it will soon be filled with other negative thinking. Instead, fill that space with the right thought, a godly thought. Lisa is a woman who did just that, and it made the difference in her life.

Forget how negative thinking affects a woman's perspective on the beauty thing. What about a woman who is just trying to survive? According to Lisa McIntire, a wife and (step, adoptive and biological) mom to five children ranging in age from 5 to 22, alleviating stinking thinking was a potential lifesaver. At age 31, when her youngest child was six months old, Lisa was diagnosed with a rare, and usually deadly, liver disease. This is what Lisa said in an interview about that difficult time in her life:

> The prognosis was dismal, so I underwent the only known medical treatment, a combination immunosuppressant and steroid drug therapy, for six months. The medication wreaked havoc on my body and the shock and stress of living with illness wounded my soul. Trying to parent four young children, work, manage mounting medical bills and maintain a marriage and household—all while facing my own seemingly imminent demise— was the most daunting challenge I have ever faced.

She didn't realize it then, but God had plans to use even this tough situation for good in her life. "Now, looking back, I can state emphatically that God has brought beauty from what I perceived as the ashes of my health and family," she said. "I can't explain exactly how He did it, or even why—except that He is Love—and I believe He wants to do the same for every hurting woman."

She credits her newfound wholeness and the discovery of her life purpose—to reach out to other hurting women with God's love and encouragement—in large part to changing her thinking. It wasn't easy in the beginning, she explains:

> For me, one of the most surprising elements of chronic illness was the constant chatter in my head that persisted long after the initial health crisis and ensuing treatment. Negative thoughts raced through my mind relentlessly, giving me very little peace and rest even though I was physically feeling better. But I knew I was going to have to take control of those negative thoughts if I wanted to get healthy and live a productive life.

So she did—by reading and meditating on God's Word and replacing her fear-filled thoughts with God's promises of unconditional love and mercy. "Now I try to start each day by spending time with God, reading and praying. That gives me the strength I need to keep my thoughts positive and hopeful instead of negative and fearful. God's in control of everything anyway, so spending my energy feeling miserable and depressed is simply a waste of the precious gift God has given me—the gift of today."

Learn from Lisa's story. What negative thoughts do you need to replace with God's promises? What specific promises can you read daily to give you hope and peace instead of negativity and fear?

## Learn to Interpret the Media

Since the media tends to have a big role in our thinking about beauty and in how we perceive ourselves, another tool in reprogramming stinkin' thinkin' is understanding how the media operates and how much it affects us when we don't fight back with godly attitudes and beliefs.

To many this won't come as a surprise, but a study in the journal *Sex Roles* found that pictures of female models can exert a powerful influence on a woman's feelings about her own body. What may surprise you is that the women in the study reacted negatively and felt badly *regardless of their own weight and size.* Researchers from the University of Missouri-Columbia (UM) measured how a group of women felt about themselves after viewing models in magazine ads for one to three minutes. In *all* cases, the women reported a drop in their level of satisfaction with their own bodies.

> "Surprisingly, we found that weight was not a factor. Viewing these pictures was just bad for everyone," said UM's Laurie Mintz. "It had been thought that women who are heavier feel worse than a thinner woman after viewing pictures of the thin ideal in the mass media. The study results do not support that theory."[6]

What the study does suggest is that trying to stop the social comparison process is important for helping all women. "Most women do not go to a counselor for advice; they look to *Seventeen* or *Glamour* magazine instead," Mintz said. "These unrealistic images of women, who are often airbrushed or partially computer-generated, have a detrimental impact on women and how they feel about themselves."[7]

Now we know (as if we didn't before) that no matter what our individual size or how much we may be perceived as beautiful by others, the media has a power over us if we let it. And the battle only gets harder as we age. Fight back by knowing how the media's projection of women and body image works.

## Understand the Media's Effect on Body Image

The popular media (television, movies, magazines) has, since World War II, increasingly held up a thinner and thinner body (and recently, ever more physically fit) as the ideal for women. If you still have any doubt about the negative effect the media has on women's self-esteem, check out these shocking statistics:

- A survey of girls 9 and 10 years old found that 40 percent have tried to lose weight, according to an ongoing study funded by the National Heart, Lung, and Blood Institute.[8]

- A 1996 study found that the amount of time adolescents spend watching soap operas, movies and music videos is directly associated with their degree of body dissatisfaction and desire to be thin.[9]

- One author reports that at age 13, 53 percent of American girls are "unhappy with their bodies." This grows to 78 percent by the time girls reach 17.[10]

- Teenage girls who viewed commercials depicting women who modeled the unrealistically thin, "ideal" type of beauty felt less confident, angrier, and more dissatisfied with their weight and appearance.[11]

As if the media blitz wasn't bad enough when it consisted only of network TV, magazines and movies, now we have to contend with the Internet, video games, cable TV and reality shows. Even the *American Idol* judges' comments about contestants' looks—think Mandisa and George Huff—have added to the fervor, turning us all into critics with high, unrealistic expectations about beauty. Who decided that the media can define beauty? Only a few decades ago, Marilyn Monroe was the pinnacle of beauty, averaging a dress size 12. Today in Hollywood, if you're not a size 0 or 2, you're considered big. Case in point: Model-turned-actress Elizabeth Hurley (rather tactlessly) said, "I'd kill myself if I was as fat as Marilyn Monroe."[12] And while it's nice that the 2008 winner of the *America's Top Model* reality show was a "plus-size" model, she wore a size 10. (I guess that means Marilyn Monroe was plus-size!)

But not everyone in Hollywood is sticking to the status quo. Some actresses, such as Kate Winslet and Jennifer Love-Hewitt, have been vocal about being themselves in spite of harsh insults from the media. Another "new" celebrity, Mandisa, from *American Idol*, became more vocal about her own self-image after being publicly picked on by Simon Cowell during the show televised to millions:

> It was a blessing in disguise. I want to live life with purpose. If [Simon] had not said anything, I don't feel I would have been as open. It has given me the opportunity to speak about it. . . . Those comments endeared me to a lot of people and the worst situation turned into the best situation. Being able to tell him I forgave him because Jesus forgave me was probably the most powerful thing I've ever done. I felt like redemption was being modeled.[13]

## Understand the Media's Motive

Unmasking the media's influence over your body image also means understanding its motivation. What is the media's motive? To make money at your expense. To do so, they are fine with not telling the truth about us. We need to call them on it and embrace the truth that no one but God defines beauty. "From Zion, perfect in beauty, God shines forth" (Ps. 50:2).

We listen to the media's lies because of our low self-esteem. If we believed in ourselves and were comfortable with our unique, God-created beauty, the media onslaught wouldn't affect us as it does. To counteract this effect, expose the lies. Learn to cut through the falsehood.

Rarely does Hollywood take a punch at its own twisted beauty images, but the 2008 movie *Penelope* did just that. More than a fairy tale, it's a commentary on how all of us should rethink what beauty is all about.

Penelope Wilhern, born to wealthy socialites, is born under the Wilhern spell, a curse that manifests itself as every girl's worst nightmare: the nose of a pig. The spell can only be broken when she finds someone to love her for who she is. So, her parents hide her away and offer a large dowry to attract suitors. Each eligible bachelor is enamored with Penelope and the cash—until they see her snout. Then they turn tail and run.

This happens again and again until Penelope declares, pig nose and all, "I like myself the way I am."

Scott Steindorff, who worked on the movie with producers Reese Witherspoon and Jennifer Simpson, said, "I call this the 'anti-Barbie' movie. Today everyone's so concerned with how they look, it's interesting to develop a story where a young woman overcomes the prejudice about her looks and proves her strength of character and eventually triumphs, finds herself, and finds true love."[14]

Maybe we're slowly moving in the right direction, but not fast enough. If we wait for Hollywood and the media to transform their ideal of beauty into a godly one, we'll be waiting forever. It's up to us to internalize God's beauty perspective by filling our minds with His thoughts.

## Detox Your Brain

Another important step in reprogramming our stinkin' thinkin' is to detox our mind. Most of us would agree wholeheartedly with the need to periodically detoxify our bodies for maximum health. But what about providing the same healthful detoxifying benefits to our brains?

### Examine What You Feed Yourself

Are you taking in too many movies and magazines instead of filling your mind with God's Word and biblical teaching? Make a list of all you watch and read in one week. How much of it is media-driven and perpetuates a negative self-image, and how much is positive, based on God's Word, positive books and wholesome television or movies, and feeds a godly self-image?

I asked my friend Lucie Costa, founder and editor of *Beautiful One* magazine and ministry, to share her thoughts on feeding the mind. In her magazine, she too helps women fight against negative self-talk. Here's what she told me:

> Word association—have you ever played that game? Someone calls out a word and you call out the first thing that comes to your mind. I used to play that game with my friends and it was always funny and interesting to hear what people associate certain words with.

Well, I'd like to share with you a word that comes to my attention daily and what I usually associate it with. Are you ready? Here's the word: *food*. And this is what I associate it with: *mind*. . . . A phrase we casually and often use makes quite a serious impact on our lives—"food for thought." What you *feed* your *mind* affects every area of your life. If you feed your mind with lies and junk, you'll start believing them, and your whole life begins to build on that foundation of deception. Lies and destructive information have the power to destroy you, but there's hope—you don't have to buy into them! You have the power within you to *choose* to change what you feed your mind! Listen, if you can choose to think negative, then you've got just as much opportunity to think positive!

What are you feeding your mind daily? Is it healthy? Is it "food" that's encouraging, inspiring, refreshing and hopeful? . . . What are your main sources of input? The phrase "Garbage in, garbage out" rings true. Have you been feeding on lies? Do you believe the best about yourself or have you allowed society, TV, magazines, even some of your friends, to dictate what you should look like, what you should own, who you should have as friends, who you should be? . . .

Have you cleaned out your refrigerator lately? Have you thrown out the food that's gone bad, that stinks? [Would you] eat that food and risk getting sick? Your mind works the same way. If you don't start cleaning out all the junk, all the rotten "food" in your mind, it's been medically proven that you will become sick (physically, mentally, emotionally and spiritually).

It's time to counteract the lies. It's time for you to accept the beautiful you that you are, inside and out, and start *believing* that you were created on purpose for a purpose here in this life! Start feeding your mind with life-giving sources![15]

Now that you've examined what you're feeding your mind, maybe it's time to go on a media fast. I was talking with Dwight Bain, a life coach who wrote the book *Destination Success*, about fasting from media input. He suggests giving up watching TV, reading magazines and viewing anything else with images that affect your mind in a negative way. Do it for 30 days and see how you feel about yourself. It may be tough at first, but you can do it.

### Actively Seek and Speak the Positive in Yourself

Seek to develop a Philippians 4:8 mindset: "Whatever is true, whatever is noble, whatever is right, whatever is pure, whatever is lovely, whatever is admirable—if anything is excellent or praiseworthy—think about such things."

We probably think twice about telling our girlfriends that they look like they've packed on the pounds, but we never hesitate to knock ourselves down. Even Solomon's wife had a hang-up because of her skin that was "darkened by the sun" (Song of Sol. 1:6), but Solomon only saw her true beauty and affirmed her with positive, uplifting words. (No wonder he had so many wives!) When it comes to words, we are the hardest on ourselves. If we could only tune our mirrors to reflect the image God sees, we would love ourselves so much more.

What you declare over your self-image has the power to make or break you. If you change the words coming out of your mouth that are toxic to your self-image, then your perception of yourself will change.

My friend Darlene Schacht, founder of Christian Women Online, wrote in her book, *The Mom Complex*: "Although I love the mall and all that fashion has to offer, when I stand on the top of life's hill, I see those styles slipping away from my grasp. And, as much as I try to cling to my youth and the beauty it holds, life pulls me over, puts a mirror in my face, and shows me beauty is fleeting." This resonates with me so much! Darlene continues, "The more I walk with God and strive to be the woman He created me to be, I see a little more of that woman in the mirror every day, and a little less of me."[16] How true, how true! Instead of fearing old age, a woman who fears the Lord is greatly to be praised (see Prov. 31:30)!

## Change How You See Yourself

- A positive outlook is part of inner beauty. Stinkin' thinkin' (that is, negativity) is not only unattractive, it can keep others from wanting to be around you. Ever seen a person that you think is beautiful, but then they open their mouth and you want to turn around? Don't let this be you.

- Learn to recognize your negative thoughts and ask yourself why you're thinking this way. What is the real, godly truth instead?

- Think on the positive things about yourself and don't compare yourself to others.

- Learn to develop a positive, godly mind.

- Magnify your best asset.

- Focus on what's next—what do you want to achieve?

- Track your progress, and pinpoint when the negativity sets in.

## An Affirmation a Day Keeps the Wrinkles Away (Somewhat!)

Every Saturday night, Stuart Smalley from *Saturday Night Live* sat in front of a mirror, looked directly at himself, and recited the same mantra: "I'm good enough, I'm smart enough, and doggone it, people like me." It may seem cheesy at first, but one way to develop positive thinking is to meditate on positive, affirming truths, particularly those from Scripture.

> *A happy heart is good medicine and a cheerful mind works healing, but a broken spirit dries up the bones.*
> (Prov. 17:22, AMP)

- There is always a way to create my destiny through God.

- The past is in the past, not in my future!

- My self-talk determines my outcome; I choose positive action steps today and every day.

- Where I am going is more important than where I am today.

- I live with passion from the King and with His direction—there are no wrong turns (though God does allow U-turns!).

- Peace is a Person, Joy is a Person, Love is a Person and that Person loves me (this is a lyric from one of my husband's songs).

- I am valuable, blessed, strong, smart and beautiful.

- Favor from the Lord is on my side.

- God has given me a sound mind; therefore, I will remove myself from any and all volatile situations or behaviors.

- I am worthy of respect and love.

- Flexible, teachable and loveable—yes, that is me!

## Meditate on Scripture

Memorize and meditate on God's truth. Here are some verses to get you started:

> "For I know the plans I have for you," declares the LORD, "plans to prosper you and not to harm you, plans to give you hope and a future" (Jer. 29:11).

> I can do everything through him who gives me strength (Phil. 4:13).

> Love the Lord God with all your passion and prayer and intelligence and energy . . . Love others as well as you love yourself. There is no commandment that ranks with these (Mark 12:30-31, *THE MESSAGE*).

> He who began a good work in you will carry it on to completion (Phil. 1:6).

> For you created my inmost being; you knit me together in my mother's womb. I praise you because I am fearfully and wonderfully made; your works are wonderful, I know that full well (Ps. 139:13-14).

## Replace Self-Doubt with Affirming Thoughts

Anxiety is closely related to our negative thoughts and feelings about ourselves. In a recent article, Dr. Linda Mintle wrote, "Negative self-talk is usually the culprit behind anxious feelings, and those negative thoughts cause us to be anxious. When we feel anxious, we see our world in a more negative light. That negative light affects our thoughts. This vicious cycle keeps anxiety going."[17]

How about changing stinkin' thinkin' into positive self-talk? Positive self-talk blocks out distractions and focuses on a positive approach to negative situations. Here are some examples to get you started; take this list and run with it. The possibilities for creating positive, powerful thoughts truly are endless!

> The greatest pollution problem we face today is negativity. Eliminate the negative attitude and believe you can do anything. Replace "If I can, I hope, maybe" with "I can, I will, I must."
> —Mary Kay Ash, Founder of Mary Kay

| Stinkin' Thinkin' | Positive Self-Talk |
| --- | --- |
| I can't. | I will. |
| What's wrong with me? | What can I learn from this? |
| That's impossible. | What is possible? All things are possible. |
| How could this have happened? | How could it be prevented next time? |
| This will never change. | How can I get past this? |
| That's just the way it is. | Whatever the problem, I'll work with it. |
| Not this again. | Things could be worse. |
| Whose fault is that? | It is what it is . . . move on. |
| That will never work. | What would work? |

Go one step further and let these words move from your mind to your mouth. Replacing the words you use will affect the way you think about yourself, and vice versa.

## Alleviate Stinkin' Stress

Stress also contributes to negative thinking, so it is extremely important to have some mental relaxation time for your overall wellbeing. Here are some simple ways to relieve mind clutter:

- Make a date with yourself (on the calendar!) for some "me" time. Go on a nature walk, scrapbook, go to the zoo or museum.

- Wake up 10 minutes earlier to make a cup of tea and pray.

- Spend time with family or friends; have a picnic or barbecue together or just hang out and do nothing.

- Sleep in on Saturday (or whatever day you can, once a week) one extra hour. When you are tired, you crave more sugary foods.

- Schedule reading time or time to learn something new; it boosts your neural connections in the brain. Try a new language, gardening or check out www.howstuffworks.com— watch and learn!

- First thing in the morning, get some fresh air; the day will go so much better.

- Get a 10-minute chair massage to relieve tension.

- Dab peppermint oil at your temples—it really works for stress.

- Sniff some aromatherapy, such as uplifting grapefruit or tangerine.

- Place some flowers at your desk or kitchen. Seeing them first thing in the morning raises enthusiasm. (Flowers don't have to be expensive; cut them from your yard or buy a bunch from the supermarket for a few dollars.)

- Eat some chicken soup; it really *is* comforting.

- Have a blue day—really. The color blue is soothing, and it won't make you crave food. (Red and yellow are known to bring on food cravings.)

- Turn your yard into a butterfly sanctuary. Go to http://livemon arch.com/free-milkweed-seeds.htm to get started.

- Losing your wallet, keys or cell phone is such a hassle and creates unnecessary stress; keep track of them by attaching a remote locator available from www.findonefindall.com.

- Getting lost when you drive is a big stress, too; get directions texted to you by calling 347-328-4667 (DIR-ECT-IONS).

## Laughter—Good for the Soul

The power of positive thinking includes learning to laugh. And besides, frowns cause wrinkles while smiles light up your face! (Thank goodness for Frownies!)

Here's a little exercise for you to try: Look in the mirror and smile (yes, it is strange, but just do it for a few minutes. Or you can do it in the car, though the guy in the car next to you may think you're crazy—but hey, you just might make him laugh! A smile is contagious you know). Now, looking in the mirror, laugh out loud. Really! It will change your mood instantly. I have done this and can promise that it works.

> The earth laughs in flowers.
> —e.e. cummings

Laughter is part of the prescription from your heavenly Father to keep you healthy, happy and steering in a positive direction. I asked Donna Schuller, Nutritional Specialist at the Crystal Cathedral Counseling Center, what she thinks about laughter being good medicine for the soul. Here's what she said:

> I like to laugh with my girlfriends. My best friend is so funny. And she's a little off-color, but you know what? I find it's just what I need, because in the ministry we deal with such serious issues so much of the time, you know. Human tragedy and human pain. I find it's really important to laugh. I love to laugh. And I like practical jokes and pull practical jokes on people. I don't like to tell jokes, I can never remember a joke. They go in one ear and out the other. But I love to have fun.

## THINKING GOD'S THOUGHTS

If we learn to think well, to cultivate mental beauty, we will develop our inner beauty and be on the path to discovering all the beauty God has placed within us. Remember Philippians 4:8—we are to think about what is *true, noble, right, pure, lovely, admirable, excellent* and *praiseworthy*. As Lucie Costa says, "Thinking this way and on these things may mean that you start *choosing* to make significant changes in your thought life. Cancel out all the negative thoughts and replace them with this new way of thinking in all areas of your life. Every time a negative or stinky thought comes into your mind, counteract it with something that's good, positive, life giving! These are tried and true ways of getting rid of your stinkin' thinkin'—once and for all!"

Just as exercise and good nutrition must become a way of life, so must positive self-talk. These days, everyone wants the quick fix, whether it's a crash diet, plastic surgery, whatever—they want instant gratification. But making a change takes time, effort and perseverance. Yeah, the old patterns will pop up in your head from time to time, but you can keep them from influencing you again. Only *you* hold the key to unlock those positive thoughts. *Turn* it, *open* up and *let them in*!

*My Cherished Daughter,*

What you think about really *does* matter!
*Remember* that My thoughts and ways are
higher than the world's trivial pursuits. I encourage
you to fix your thoughts on things that really count.
Focus on anything that is good *and right.*
Reflect on the pure and lovely. Let your thoughts pass
the *praiseworthy* test. But remember, knowledge
isn't enough. Putting My thoughts into practice is
what leads to *true peace.* As you refocus, remember
that I'm for you today and always. You can be totally
confident that I'll faithfully complete the beautiful
work *I've birthed* in you!

Thinking good thoughts of you,
Your Heavenly *Father*

Proverbs 23:7; Isaiah 55:9; Philippians 4:8-9; 1:6; Psalm 139:17

(by LeAnn Weiss-Rupard)

# Twelve

# Jealousy: Beauty Turned Beast

D o you remember the famous shampoo commercial featuring Kelly Lebrock, known for her famous, seemingly vain, words, "Don't hate me because I'm beautiful"? Well, we shouldn't hate her because she's beautiful and we shouldn't judge her, either. I saw her once in an interview and she said she felt funny saying the oh-so-familiar line, but it paid the mortgage.

Supermodel Kim Alexis once revealed that she felt uncomfortable about dressing up a little before going out, in fear of being judged for "looking good." Her husband would say, "Are you going out like that? Shouldn't you put something else on or a little makeup?" Now she feels comfortable enough to dress up or dress down without any distractions, because she's confident that her value comes from God.

Both models were aware that others might see them and be jealous. I once read in

> A calm and undisturbed mind and heart are the life and health of the body, but envy, jealousy, and wrath are like rottenness of the bones.
>
> —Proverbs 14:30, AMP

an article that the word "jealousy" stems from the French root *jaloux*, itself a relative of the low-Latin word *zelosus* (full of zeal). Here's where it gets a little more interesting: *Zelosus* has its roots in the Greek verb that means "to boil," ferment, or yeast. I guess it is true; we boil when we feel jealous or envious of other women that have "more beauty" than we do. (I bet some of us would like for that yeast to be planted right below the breast plate and let it "rise," fermenting away some of the fat from those thighs. But seriously . . .)

Jealousy overlaps envy; we can experience both at the same time. The philosopher John Rawls distinguished between jealousy and envy. He suggested that jealousy involves the wish to "keep" what one has, and envy means to "get" what one does not have. Either one can lead to feelings of inferiority. Though we'd like to somehow "blame" other women for making us feel inferior, it really all comes down to being comfortable in our own skin. Why do we judge others, and more particularly, why are we so jealous of other women? Maybe it's our competitive culture or the constant media onslaught of beautiful, stick-thin, just-about-perfect movie stars and supermodels. Maybe it's just ingrained in our female nature. Whatever the reason, we tend to constantly compare ourselves to others and strive to be something else, something different, something perfect. This comparison trap can quickly turn into gossip, envy and jealousy—none of which are beautiful.

## COMPARISON: THE ROOT OF ALL FEELINGS OF INFERIORITY

We've all encountered jealousy at one time or another. Either we've envied someone, or we've been the object of someone else's jealousy. My first memory of jealousy dates back to when my dad remarried. He was 35 and his new wife was 21, and she had two kids ages 2 and 4. My sister and I were 10 and 13. Dad's new wife tended to manipulate his affections, issuing ultimatums because of his love for my sister and me. I was never allowed to be alone with my dad after the marriage. No more lunch dates, no more "Daddy's little girl," because his wife got upset and claimed that he loved us more than her. She monitored our phone calls and sometimes even took away the receiver. It wasn't always bad—we even enjoyed some good times when her guard was down—but she drove a wedge between my dad and me because of her jealousy.

I lost my father to the evils of jealousy. Even up to the day he died, my stepmother wouldn't let me talk to him. As he was on his deathbed (I was in Florida; he was in Connecticut), my cousin intervened on his end and grabbed the phone from her so that I could to tell my dad how sorry I was for the many mistakes I'd made in the past and that I loved him. He said, "I love you, Shell," in a weak, muzzled voice under his oxygen mask. My sister and I flew up north to say goodbye, and Dad managed to stay alive for three more days. Though my stepmother seemed okay upon our arrival, a few days after he died, she told me that he didn't think I was his daughter. Can you imagine the pain I felt? I died a thousand deaths as I sat across from her. I thought to myself, *I am a Christian now, so how do I handle this? Maybe I will put my Christlike behavior on the back burner and knock her out, then ask for forgiveness.* I responded by pointing out that I looked just like my father. She answered, "A lot of people look like other people." I was shocked, and I knew I was no match for the venom stemming from her bitterness and insecurity. At his funeral, she had the nerve to tell me that someone had asked who I was. When they found out I was my father's daughter, they said my stepmother was too young-looking and thought we were the same age. More words of jealousy.

As tears roll down my face while writing this, I realize this is the first time I have put this part of my story into words, even though it has been four years since my dad died. Telling it brings the reality crashing in: He is gone. And my last memories of my dad are filled with the painful reminders of the ugliness of jealousy.

## THE OUTCOME OF JEALOUSY

As I have been, all of us can be affected for years by the jealous words and actions of others. Do women, young or old, really understand the outcome of jealousy? Do we realize how long the sting of ungodly, unbeautiful, envious words and actions last in the heart of their victim?

When I watched the 1998 movie *Ever After, A Cinderella Story* with Drew Barrymore, I related to her character, Danielle, in so many ways. Danielle lost her father at the age of eight (I lost mine when he remarried); she disguised herself as royalty (I hid my past to my boyfriend, now husband); and we shared a passion for books and the experience of a controlling stepmother. Danielle's perceptive question to the baroness could have been written for me: "What bothers you more, stepmother? That I am common or that I am competition?" Competition is big with women, and it is different than the competition between men.

In high school I was outgoing, but being from a single-parent family, I didn't quite fit in or have the designer clothes and expensive house that the "popular" girls had. We lived in an apartment with my mom when I was not with my dad, and we moved a lot. I began to want what these girls had. I remember being envious of the cheerleaders in particular, the girls who seemed to have the best of everything, including the cute guys. Although those same guys thought I was "cute" and seemed to like my fun personality, it was never enough for a date. I couldn't compete with the cheerleaders and their alligator-logo shirts (I know I'm dating myself). So instead, I acted on my jealous impulses and decided that I would win these guys in other ways: I would compromise my values and see them behind their girlfriends' backs—which only fueled the jealousy and insecurity. I was looking for attention any way I could get it, but my methods backfired and caused a lot of pain and led to years of counseling.

High school memories faded, but that wasn't the last time I confronted jealousy—this time as the object. I rededicated myself to Christ when I was 26, and a short time later, I became engaged to my husband, Angelo. During our engagement, I attended a large Bible study of about a thousand people, where Angelo was a worship leader. One particular night I sat down in a seat before the worship began. I wore a hat, so I wasn't recognizable from the back. Two girls sat down a row back and began to talk about Angelo and how he wasn't married yet so he was still open for business. Plus, they were certain we would break up and one of them would "get" him away from me. I felt anger, for sure, but more than that, I was appalled at the jealousy from other Christian women toward me.

In her bestselling book *Battlefield of the Mind*, Joyce Meyer had this to say about jealousy:

> Vine's *An Expository Dictionary of New Testament Words* defines the Greek word translated *envy* as "the feeling of displeasure produced by witnessing or hearing of the advantage or prosperity of others." *Jealousy* is defined by Webster as "feelings of envy, apprehension, or bitterness." I interpret this definition as being fearful of losing what you have to another; resentment of another's success, arising from feelings of envy.
>
> Envy will cause a person to behave in a way that is callous and crude—even animalistic at times. Envy caused Joseph's brothers to sell him into slavery. They hated him because their father loved him so much.[1]

## ALL SHAPES, SIZES AND OBJECTS

Jealousy and envy aren't limited to our feelings about other women. These mental attitudes raise their ugly heads toward a variety of subjects. I am not proud to admit this, but I have been jealous on occasion of the churches where my husband has lead worship. My list of grievances? Too much time with the band, holidays automatically committed for church "programs," vacations cut short, too many phone calls, paychecks under market value. To top it off, I've felt certain that people were envious of me. At times I wouldn't even attend church, feeling angry and resentful of his calling. Then there were the tantrums at home and the way my jealousy showed on my face at church. Believe me, I'm not proud of my childish, jealous behavior.

Perhaps your husband or parent spent too much time away from you (or so you thought), giving you "cause" for your own pity party. In my case, I finally dug deep into my heart and asked for forgiveness. God had called Angelo to help His people enter into the throne room of heaven through worship, and I, selfish Shelly, wanted him all to myself. So there you have it: I am human and a spoiled brat. Yet over the years, I have learned to accept what Angelo does and I'm happy to tell you how proud I am of him and the sacrifices he has made to bring glory to God.

## WHY DO WE GET JEALOUS?

So where does the ugly beast originate? What causes us to feel so strongly that someone else has an attribute or possession we should have? Or that someone wants something we have, so we turn jealous to protect what we "own"? Jealousy and envy rear their ugly heads for many reasons, but the roots are insecurity, pride and an unhealthy self-focus. I have heard it be said that jealousy can originate from facts, thoughts, perceptions and memories, but also imagination, guessing and assumptions.

Maybe for you it started in childhood when you competed with your sister, who was prettier or made better grades than you. Jealousy begins in a place of insecurity, but it grows when it's fed with pride, selfishness or even materialism.

It doesn't seem to matter how "successful" a woman is, either. Jealousy affects us all. Author, speaker, television cohost and singer Michelle McKinney Hammond admits to struggling with jealousy:

> I find that I'm jealous when I'm not happy with how my life is going. But instead of focusing on how to make my life go the way I want it to, I start looking around me at what everybody else is doing. All that energy would be better spent if I'd focus on what it is about my life that I don't like. There is something I can do about my today every day. And so can you. Learn to walk through every day with grace and be able to celebrate what's going on with others.[2]

Anita Renfroe adds to that by saying she ignores jealousy in others: "It is a spiritual problem in the heart of the person who is jealous, and there's pretty much nothing you can do to stop it in others. When I feel it rising up in me, I am aware that the root is always pride and a sense of entitlement, both of which are cause to hit my knees and begin to say a long list of 'Thank Yous' to my Father—a spirit of gratitude and a spirit of jealousy cannot coexist."[3]

"Jealousy is a Pandora's box. James 3:16 says, 'Where jealousy and selfish ambition exist, there is disorder and every evil thing.' Open the door to jealousy and other evils will follow."[4] We must learn to recognize it for the negative force it is and the causes behind it, both in others and in ourselves.

## ACCEPT IT, LET IT GO, GIVE IT TO GOD

The only way to truly deal with jealousy is to accept your feelings first. Stop fighting it and surrender. Observe the feelings without judgment and ask God to remove the thorn. Jealousy is like a weed; you cannot tolerate it in the garden of your life, or it will grow and choke out the good things God is trying to cultivate in you. If you allow it, jealousy will destroy relationships and wreak havoc in every area of your life. You know it's gonna come up again, so don't condemn yourself; keep surrendering the feeling.

"God opposes the proud but *gives grace* to the *humble*" (Jas. 4:6, emphasis added). Fight jealousy and envy by learning to cultivate a humble heart and attitude. Humility does not mean thinking less of yourself; it only means thinking of yourself less. Pride is at the heart of a jealous attitude and humility is the only antidote.

Seeing ourselves as God sees us and not comparing ourselves to others will also smother jealousy. Sounds simple, right? It is simple, but it isn't easy. Allow yourself to view your accomplishments, appreciate what you have and compare yourself *to yourself*. We can't love others if we don't love ourselves. The key to loving and accepting yourself is learning to say and believe, "I am unique and wonderfully made by God, who loves me and cherishes me just as I am."

I recently spoke with Abigail Mason, who starred in *Saving Sarah Cain*. When we spoke, she was filming in Canada for the movie *Jake's Run*. About her sense of being created by God, she explained, "I am unique and

I love that I am so unique. I think beauty is defined by being different, uniquely designed by God. In L.A., people use the 'cookie-cutter blonde' term a lot, so I've learned that you should embrace your unique differences, abilities and gifts."[5]

This passage from Psalm 139 is one of the most poignant reminders in Scripture of how intimately God knows and cherishes you and has uniquely created you. Take a beauty breather and soak in God's profound love for you as you read David's words:

> Oh yes, you shaped me first inside, then out;
> you formed me in my mother's womb.
> I thank you, High God—you're breathtaking!
> Body and soul, I am marvelously made!
> I worship in adoration—what a creation!
> You know me inside and out,
> you know every bone in my body;
> You know exactly how I was made, bit by bit,
> how I was sculpted from nothing into something.
> Like an open book, you watched me grow from conception to birth;
> all the stages of my life were spread out before you,
> The days of my life all prepared
> before I'd even lived one day
> (Ps. 139:13-16, *THE MESSAGE*).

As you spend time praying and reading God's Word, the Spirit will guide you, and slowly but surely your feelings of jealousy and envy will fade. In Galatians 5:22-26, Paul shows us what this looks like: "But the fruit of the Spirit is love, joy, peace, patience, kindness, goodness, faithfulness, gentleness and self-control. Against such things there is no law. Let us not become conceited, provoking and envying each other." In other words, this is the way we should behave when we are living by the Spirit instead of by the "flesh," which is controlled by our earthly desires, including jealousy.

Self-control is another important key to ridding our lives of the green-eyed monster. It takes patience and diligence to overcome a pattern of harmful thinking. Spiritual maturity is a process, but we have God's assurance that He will walk through it with us, and that every time we fall, He will be there to pick us up and point us in the right direction.

## OVERCOMING THE BEAST

*Don't hit back; discover beauty in everyone.*
*If you've got it in you, get along with everybody.*
*Don't insist on getting even; that's not for you to do.*
*"I'll do the judging," says God. "I'll take care of it."*
*Our Scriptures tell us that if you see your enemy hungry,*
*go buy that person lunch, or if he's thirsty, get him a drink.*
*Your generosity will surprise him with goodness.*
*Don't let evil get the best of you;*
*get the best of evil by doing good.*
—Romans 12:17-21, *THE MESSAGE*

You can live a life filled with beauty instead of jealousy, though our human nature wants to go the other way. Seek to be more like Christ, exercise self-control and fill your mind with the good, the godly and the truly beautiful. In addition to reading God's Word, here are some more ways to overcome the jealousy monster.

### Tips for Overcoming Jealousy

- *Love, love, love.* Love your enemies and love your neighbors. Easier said than done, I know. But it goes back to letting go of control and letting God control. You can choose to be loving, gracious and kind in *any* situation.

- *Be content with what you have, and don't try to keep up with the Joneses.* Trust that God will bring the blessings He wants for you into your life and be happy for the way He blesses other people. He has a unique plan for you that does not mirror the plan He has for anyone else. Your friend bought a Gucci bag. So what? Don't run to the department store to even things up. Materialism is a close cousin of jealousy and can become a monster of its own (massive credit card debt included).

- *Have compassion for others and try to see things through their eyes.* Everyone fights battles and carries burdens that aren't necessarily apparent; only God truly knows the depths of another person's heart. Hurting people hurt others, so give her the benefit of the doubt. Even if she's just having a bad day, everyone deserves a break.

- *Show mercy and grace to the people in your path.* Mercy is not getting what we deserve; grace is getting the good that we *don't* deserve.

- *Refuse to gossip.* "The words of a gossip are like choice morsels; they go down to a man's inmost parts" (Prov. 18:8). Nothing good comes from idle chatter, so avoid situations when you'll be tempted. If there is a certain person or group of people who tend toward gossip in conversation, stay away from them or kindly tell them you're on a "tongue fast"—maybe they'll join you.

- *Face your shortcomings and take action to correct them.* If your jealousy uncovers something you need to change, don't blame or criticize others. Instead, work on what you need to change. For example, if you're jealous of someone who is physically fit, start a healthier eating plan or join a gym. When you take responsibility for yourself, you will find that you are not as jealous of others.

- *Find common ground with other women.* You may not have the same background or be in the same life situation, but if you try, you can almost always make a connection. Do you both have kids? Maybe you both like to scrapbook, hike or bake. Have you read an interesting book or seen a good movie lately? Strike up a conversation; it will help you look past your differences with others and celebrate common bonds.

- *Be humble, find ways to serve and show kindness to others.* Pray and ask God to show you people or situations that need a helping hand or a healing touch. You can babysit for a single mom, take cookies to an elderly neighbor or deliver balloons to a children's hospital. These things might seem small, but each act of kindness will take you closer to the goal of getting your mind off yourself (bye-bye jealousy!) and showing God's love to others.

## REPLACE JEALOUSY WITH JOY

At the age of 15, author, speaker and singer Jennifer Rothschild was diagnosed with a rare, degenerative eye disease that eventually stole her sight. Because of the blindness, her dreams of becoming a commercial artist and cartoonist faded, but words and music have replaced her canvas and palette for more than 25 years. She offers these words of wisdom for constructively dealing with jealousy toward a friend.

If you're experiencing jealousy, it may be a reflection of your own insecurity. First, if you want to overcome it, begin targeting those places where you feel jealous and compliment your friend in those areas. If she has a really nice figure, compliment her about that. Then you're turning your envy into encouragement. A second

> Good thoughts and actions can never produce bad results; bad thoughts and actions can never produce good results. This is but saying that nothing can come from corn but corn, nothing from nettles but nettles.
> —James Allen, *As a Man Thinketh*

way to handle jealousy is to thank God for your friend. Then thank God for your good qualities, because you've got just as many as she does. The more you do this, the more your insecurity will wane.[6]

You will break free from the chains of jealousy and its ugly twin, envy, when you overcome insecurity, low self-esteem, low self-worth and pain from the past. As a woman created with true beauty, you are free to be all God wants you to be! Go now and paint your lips with words of encouragement and let your positive affirmations reflect kindness, inspiring others to love their own uniqueness that lies within.

*My Beautiful Daughter,*

*Do your best and avoid the comparison trap!*
*Take pride in yourself and don't worry about*
*what others have. Jealousy and quarreling is worldly.*
*But love is patient and kind and does not envy.*
*Focus on your motives. Be still before Me*
*and wait patiently for Me. Choose to celebrate*
*when you feel inferior, weak, insulted, persecuted,*
*or if you're experiencing hard times. In your humility,*
*you'll experience My perfect power. You'll find*
*that godliness mixed with contentment leads*
*to a big bonus. Be grateful for what I've*
*already given you. I'll make your life*
*fall in pleasant places.*

*Building you up,*
*Your heavenly Father*

Galatians 6:3-5; 1 Corinthians 3:3; 13:4; Psalm 37:7;
2 Corinthians 12:9-10; 1 Timothy 6:6-8; Psalm 16:6

(By LeAnn Weiss-Rupard)

# Thirteen

## Discover Your Passion Pathway

I can remember when I first discovered my passion for writing *Beauty by God*. I told my husband, Angelo, how I wished there were a book "out there" that discussed beauty and balance from a biblical standpoint, combined with an informative holistic approach to life without a bunch of mystical stuff added. Then I half-joked, "I want to write that book." He became fully supportive of my launch into the book world. As I began to pursue this writing adventure with a toddler and a five-year-old, everything you can imagine happened along the way. Before I tell you about the journey, I have to say that I would not be able to pursue my passions without my faith, family and friends. Some of the amazing activities in this chapter (such as the Passion Pathway Party) helped me to get to the next level and get a handle on tough situations.

In the space of a few years, six of my immediate family members went to be with the Lord: my dad, my husband's parents, both of my grandmothers and my beautiful cousin. I almost did not make it myself when I got pneumonia and landed in the hospital for several days. Besides homeschooling my kids, being part of the worship team and trying to be a good wife, I wasn't sure the dream of this book would ever become a reality.

I am not asking for violins to play; I'm only telling you this to illustrate that in spite of everything that could have discouraged me on this writing project, I never gave up. Okay, so there were times when I did not want to get out of bed—but I kept pressing on. Passion burned in me, and I believe it was embedded in my heart by God Himself.

Oh, I'd felt passion in the past. But my passion ignited but never stayed lit. Like being an artist, for instance: I was accepted to Pratt Art School in New York City, but I didn't go because a guy got in the way. I wanted to be an actress and even appeared on *One Life to Live,* but I didn't move ahead because a guy got in the way. In my second year of college, earning a degree in graphic arts, I left and didn't finish because a guy got in the way.

With my husband's support, I finally began to act and follow through on my passions—established a mural painting business, became an esthetician and herbalist, raising my children, singing on the worship team and launching a writing career. A guy got in the way! It worked in my favor this time, because I was following God.

## PASSION IS BEAUTIFUL

My dictionary lists several definitions of "passion":

- the sufferings of Christ between the night of the Last Supper and His death
- intense, driving or overmastering feeling or conviction
- an outbreak of anger
- ardent affection
- a strong liking or desire for or devotion to some activity, object or concept
- sexual desire
- an object of desire or deep interest

Interesting, isn't it, that the first definition of the word "passion" describes what Jesus did for you and me. He lived to die, and His passion was to suffer for sinners. His suffering was horrific on the outside, but never has the world seen a more beautiful outcome than Jesus' demonstration of sacrifice and love. In Isaiah 53:2, the Bible says that Jesus had "no beauty or majesty to attract us to him, nothing in his appearance that we should desire Him." In other words, His physical appearance did not make Him beautiful, but His glorious beauty shone in everything He did.

In strong contrast, the world's definition of *passion* usually revolves around a sexual desire or a strong devotion to objects. Everywhere you look, the word "sex" is related to lipstick, shampoo, clothes, food, beverages and even cell phones—it's all about sex, *sex* and more SEX. I guess you can say I am a bit tired of the word used inappropriately—so tired that I don't even want to look sexy (except for my husband's eyes alone . . . sometimes . . . well, no, 'cause he will chase me around the house! Just kidding). When I go out, I want to look good, but my goodness, aren't we all over the abuse of the word "sex"?!

## WHAT KEEPS US FROM OUR PASSION?

Despite the world's misunderstanding of passion, we can't let our culture steal such a wonderful word away from us. We must discover and pursue the godly passions placed within us. Passion is an integral part of whole-person beauty, but all too often, it gets buried or snuffed out. So how do we ignite it? One way is to refocus. My good friend Amber Buckley believes that "passion requires focus, and if you are trying to be a jack-of-all-trades, your passion can be squelched. How can you be passionate when in survival mode? So set realistic goals or end up frustrated with unachieved expectations."[1]

### Frustration and Discouragement

When I start to feel my passion deflate, it's usually because I've either put too much on my plate or not enough (usually it's way too much). When that happens, I need to readjust my time, schedule or priorities. I also tend to overanalyze my circumstance or rerun the tape of negative thoughts in my mind. I've learned to recognize where they are coming from . . . and it's not from God. You probably hear these tapes, too. Maybe you have said to yourself, *I always mess up. I'll never be good at anything*, or *I'm too old, too young, too tall, too short, too this, too that, blah blah blah . . .* (we all play that tape, don't we?).

Late one night while writing this chapter, I thought, *I am too pooped to even write anything else on passion*, and was about to turn off the TV (I had muted the sound) and go to sleep. Just then, I became intrigued by a guest on *The Glenn Beck Show*. I saw the name at the bottom of the screen: Christopher Gardner, who wrote the book *The Pursuit of Happyness* (the movie starring Will Smith was inspired by Gardner's story). So I turned up the volume and was immediately inspired; this man mentioned passion in every other sentence! More than 20 years ago, he was homeless, raising his son after the mother of his child left them, and working a full-time job. Gardner said, "You've got to be bold enough to get it. . . . Passion, it can't be bought, it can't be taught, and Harvard can't teach it to you. Passion, you've got to have it!"

He should know. After watching a man pull up in a Ferrari on the street, he asked him, "What do you do and how do you do it?" The man replied, "I am a stockbroker." With that answer, passion suddenly burned inside of Gardner, not for materialism but for a way out from living on the streets and in subway stations. In a different interview, his son was asked, "What do you remember about living on the streets?" His reply? "Every time I looked up, I saw my father was there." Wow, that brought me to tears. What dedication and passion Christopher Gardner had for his family. He even won the 2002 Father of the Year award. *That* is passion, if I ever saw it.

> When you **spread the joy** of an authentic passionate life in God to **others**, it brings further glory to God, and it **increases your** own joy when, like the image in a mirror, it is **reflected** back to you.
> —John Avant, *The Passion Promise*[2]

Living in the middle of difficult or painful circumstances, like Gardner's, can either extinguish the passion fire in us or keep it alive in our hearts. Take a look at your passion and figure out if circumstances or negative thoughts have consumed your determination or motivated you to pursue it even harder.

## Baggage

On the other hand, you may think, *Why bother to dream? Nothing ever works out for me.* As soon as that thought tries to sneak in, take hold of it and say, *No. That's not true. The truth is, God created me for a purpose and He has promised to give me hope and a future.*

Try not to let your mind be a trash dump anymore. Let God's truths about you penetrate your mind and fan the flame of passion in your life. He is the Author of passion!

You know we've *all* messed up, humiliated ourselves, sold ourselves short, dishonored God and our families, chased after things that are worthless and eaten the bitter fruit of our terrible choices. Whether your childhood was tragic or you grew up in a bubble, you're still human. You've blown it. It's okay. Ask for God's forgiveness, then put the baggage down and leave it in the past.

Maybe your baggage cart is loaded with guilt about sexual promiscuity or lies you've told. Or maybe you've packed a few suitcases with shame because of past physical or sexual abuse. Do you carry a backpack full of fear that someone will find out that you're deeply in debt or that you have an eating disorder? What about this ball and chain: addiction to alcohol, food, drugs, sex, whatever? It's a heavy load, isn't it? I know, because I've carried it around with me, too. When I first met Angelo, I thought, *Please, don't let anyone tell him that I bartended and lived immorally, even lived a double life.* All he knew about me was that my grandmother and uncle owned a popular local Christian book and music store. Little did he know that I was popular in another type of customer service store—at the bar where I used to work.

So what do you and I do with this lifelong cart of baggage? Hold on to the bags in order to get neckaches, heartaches and bellyaches (oh, I did) from the stress of holding on to it all? No. We can stop dragging all that around, unload the cart and let God replace it with passion for Him and His purposes for our lives.

You don't need to live in the past. The past ended one second ago and God has a plan for your life (see Jer. 29:11). Brick upon brick, stone upon stone, you are becoming stronger, because the mortar God is using is the knowledge that you are wonderfully and fearfully made!

## Fear

Fear is another surefire passion thief. The *Random House Dictionary* defines "fear" as "a distressing emotion aroused by impending danger, evil, pain, etc., *whether the threat is real or imagined*; the feeling or condition of being afraid" (emphasis added). What are you afraid of? Failure? Success? Other people's opinions? Rejection? Whatever it is, if you let fear control you, true passion will be hard to come by. Fear whispers, "That's pretty risky. You'd better not try," and "What if people think you're crazy? It's safer here in your comfort zone." Don't listen! I've heard it said that *fear* stands for False Evidence Appearing Real. Fear is a feeling, nothing more and nothing less. But you don't have to live by feelings. By a sheer act of will, you can pursue your dreams even when you're afraid.

In her book *Feel the Fear and Do It Anyway*, Susan Jeffers offers this encouragement from her own experience: "As I began to do things on my own, I began to taste the deliciousness of an emerging self-confidence. It wasn't all comfortable—in fact, a lot of it was extremely uncomfortable. I felt like a child learning to walk and falling frequently. But with each step I felt a little surer of my ability to handle my life."[3]

When I had my first son, Angelo Jr., he arrived a month early and I experienced some complications. Angelo Jr. was born with red hair, blue eyes and very pale skin. I thought it was normal for a baby to have such pale skin, but when the nurses came in and took him to the NICU, I did what I do best—panic. The next day when I visited my little newborn, I could not touch him too much; the nurses said that doing so would overstimulate him. All the doctors knew at that point was that Angelo Jr. needed a blood transfusion and had low blood sugar, but they told us the worst possibilities first—that it could be leukemia or a bone marrow disease. All I could think was, *My son is not in my arms and I want him now.*

Just as I got back to my room, the phone rang. It was Marie Kuck, a friend of my husband's whom I had not met, whose son was a year old and had a rare undiagnosed syndrome. She prayed with me and encouraged me with words about her own horrific circumstances. She also said something that has stuck with me for years: "God will heal Angelo Jr., I know He will, Shelly!" God healed her son, Nathaniel, in heaven, when he was four and a half. Marie is an extremely selfless woman and now brings hope to many families with ill children through the foundation Nathaniel's Hope. She often counsels others with this motto: "Sometimes tragedy can bring passion for a cause that can bring triumph." Marie helped bring me hope in a trying time, and I began to see how great passion can arise out of fear.

On Angelo Jr.'s third day in the NICU, we met a woman whose daughter was born not only with a tumor on her brain but also addicted to crack. The mother, grandmother and brother were all crying outside the room, and my husband asked if he could pray with them. This mother looked up and said yes. He wanted to know if the family had a relationship with Christ, and they said no. "Do you want to know Him?" Angelo asked, and all three together exclaimed, "Yes!" We stood in a circle and prayed as they cried and asked the Lord into their hearts. The next day, back at the NICU, the baby's tumor was gone. As the family hugged Angelo and thanked him, he replied, "That is the power of prayer and the power of God—a bad situation turned into triumph!" God's purpose in our difficult experience with Angelo Jr. spilled over into another family's life and brought them both physical and spiritual healing.

For the next year and a half, three times a week, I took my son to Nemours Clinic for blood work. Each visit, I sat in the waiting room and prayed for the other kids and parents, knowing that their situations were much worse than ours; Angelo Jr. had been diagnosed with thalasemia minor, a blood disorder (we have not had to have his blood work done in several years). Before my son came along, I already had an interest in homeopathic medicines and had studied them here and there, but our difficult circumstances with him stirred up passion in me for the health of my family. I knew I would end up practicing alternative medicine further down the road.

What experiences in your life—difficult or exhilarating—have brought an opportunity to increase your passion for either a new or existing cause? God desires to fuel the fire of hope in your heart and use it to fulfill the purposes He created for you long before you were born. Let the passion rise in yourself so that it can spill over into other people's lives and circumstances.

## PASSION CHALLENGE

You may experience roadblocks to passion, but once you've put those obstacles behind you, it's time to move toward your passion. Rather than reciting general principles about how to rediscover passion in your life, I'd like to show you an exercise that will help you examine the true desires of your heart. In order to do this exercise, you'll need to set aside some time alone to fully explore your hidden passions. Carve out at least an hour (a half-day would be even better) and follow these steps:

1. Get quiet with God. Find a place of solitude in your home, or somewhere else, and just be still. Turn off the TV, computer and cell phone. Make yourself and this time of reflection a priority. Be comfortable and surround yourself with beautiful things, such as beeswax or soy candles, essential oils, a beautiful view or a fountain to quiet your mind and heart and delight your senses. Put on your most comfortable clothes, grab a cozy throw, prop yourself up with fluffy pillows and turn on some relaxing music.

2. Pour yourself some fresh, cold water and prepare a plate of healthful "brain food" snacks such as raw almonds or fresh fruit. Now you're ready to reflect.

3. Have your Bible and/or an inspirational book, and a pen and journal (a spiral-bound notebook will do) on hand to capture your thoughts and prayers.

4. Think forward and backward. Don't be afraid. You're not going to dwell on the past, but it's part of who you are, so it's important to include some memories in this retreat. Just take it one

step at a time. Begin with a travel back through your childhood and adolescence. What memories do you have of passion being ignited? What did you want to be when you grew up? Where did you spend your free time? What made you feel so happy you thought you might burst? Gather some photographs and other mementos to help you remember what it was like to freely follow your passions.

Fast forward to now. Ask yourself these questions:

> *If I didn't have to do it perfectly I would try . . .*
> *If money were no object I would . . .*

Such thoughts might seem insignificant in the big scheme of your life, but anything that captures your attention or makes your heart beat faster provides a clue to your God-given passions. Write your thoughts in your journal and ask God to give you more insight into what makes you tick.

After this reflective time, don't put aside your written thoughts and forget them. Begin to look for opportunities to pursue your passion. Take time to think and pray about how to fuel and grow your passion in godly ways. Thank God for His guidance as He helps you find and walk down your passion pathway. Remember to put yourself in everything you create. *Passion is . . .*

P ossible—Believe that all things are possible with God.

A cts—Act on your desires and don't procrastinate.

S timulating—Awaken your mind and senses with reading, art or music.

S uccess—Apply yourself and reap the rewards.

I nspired—Surround yourself with people, places and objects that ignite you.

O bservation—Look closely at opportunities, talented people and those you admire.

N urturing—Cultivate the artist within.

## Find a Focus Partner

We should never travel through life alone. Sometimes we need someone besides our spouse or family to help us keep our focus on the passions of our lives. My friend Leslie is not only my "focus partner," she's also my prayer partner. Here's how we help one another stay focused on our passions. You and your partner can adapt your own format; however, this works for us.

- First, take the Motivational DNA™ test by Tamara Lowe (find it at www.getmotivatedbook.com/Test.aspx). Tamara says that people are motivated by five things: production, connection, stability, variety or awards—internal or external. Most of us are challenged by at least three of the five. Remember that motivation is a mindset; it can be learned.

- Pick a goal—short-term or long-term—that is attainable (Leslie and I pick three).

- Set a reasonable date. (For instance, if you want to be an illustrator, you could sign up for art classes or check out the local college programs, internships, and so on. I knew I wanted to write a book, so I went to various places to become an expert on my subject of passion, including writer's conferences, a speaker's academy and health seminars, and read hundreds of books on the topics found in *Beauty by God*. It sounds like a lot of work, but my goal was big, and knew I had the support to attain my five-year plan.)

- Meet once a month or so, by telephone or in person. Each person gets 30 minutes to talk about her or his progress (or lack thereof). The first five minutes, talk about what you did or did not do with your goals and where you might be stuck.

- Brainstorm together: Give each other ideas and feedback about what else you can do or connections to someone who can help (if you are together, use Play-doh, scented markers and silly toys to bring out your creativity).

- The last five minutes: Discuss what's next and bring forth new goals.

Once you both know what you are doing, bring in another person. Now you're ready for the Passion Pathway Party.

## PASSION PATHWAY PARTY

Everyone should take the Motivational DNA test before the party.

- Invite like-minded friends. Be sure to tell them what kind of party it is and that, no, you are not selling anything from a direct marketing company.

- Invite as many as 20 and tell them to bring food from the list you will provide for them. As your guests arrive, congregate near the kitchen, as this will keep the mood informal and appetites satisfied.

- Start with a prayer for guidance, healing, humility, courage, financial breakthroughs, new ministries and for God to lead the way, as He wants to give us the desires of our hearts (see Ps. 37:4).

- Have plenty of trade, travel, fashion or home magazines on hand, as well as inspirational quotes or favorite books that ignited your passion, and art pieces or photography of beautiful places around the globe.

- Provide plenty of pads, pencils, scented markers, Play-doh and silly toys to inspire brainstorming. Let one person begin by saying, "I always wanted to . . ." or "I find this gets in the way every time I . . ." Try to complete these sentence with action plans for moving forward or overcoming specific obstacles. Each person should get a turn of 5 to 10 minutes (longer if only four to six people are at the party). Choose someone to be "the timer," or these parties can last all night. Any longer than two to three hours will exhaust rather than excite.

- Network together. We all have connections. I have a couple of friends I call "great connectors"—Torry Martin and LeAnn Weiss. I can't believe how many people they connect others to, fulfilling friends' passions. (That's what I'm gonna call them: The Passion Connectors.) These connections don't have to be grandiose; they can be as simple as a neighbor who loves to bake or a friend at church who's been wanting to start a new ministry.

- Make a personal sign. Pick one of your passions and write it at the top of a piece of paper, then write out a few things that need to happen to get where you want to go. (Please don't misunderstand me: I am not talking about the "law of attraction" that you may have heard about. I am recommending that you write down your best understanding of the steps needed to fulfill your dream.) After you are done, make sure to post your list where you will see it every day. By doing this, you have applied action, which keeps your attention engaged and motivated toward your passion pathway.

- Give guests a "passion goody bag" filled with affirmations such as:

> *It is my job to do the work, not judge the work.*
> *Dear God, I will take care of the quantity.*
> *You take care of the quality.*
>
> —Julia Cameron, *The Artist Within*

> *Passion is the first step to achievement—*
> *your desire determines your destiny.*
> *The stronger your fire, the greater the desire,*
> *and the greater the potential.*
>
> —John Maxwell

• Plan the next time to meet. If everyone's schedules are too full to throw another party, plan a webinar or a teleconference. (Try www.freeconference.com.) Maybe you can plan for four physical parties a year and do the rest through the Internet.

If we take the time to help each other discover and pursue the passions God has placed within all of us, we will find greater excitement and motivation to stay on our passion pathway. Passion Pathway Parties are a great way to ignite and fuel passions, as well as create accountability and partnerships for the journey.

CC (a.k.a. Colleen Curtis) saw a need for this kind of community and started Firepit Friday, a podcast that brings together musical artists from around the world to discuss the creative process and their experiences, as well as to make connections with other artists. CC said, "By creating Firepit Friday the podcast, I feel like it's my time to give back. I get to take the gifts that God has given to me and apply them to helping other people make their dreams come true. The benefits of bonding with the people I interview are what makes life good!"[4]

## LIVING LIFE WITH PASSION

What does it look like to live your life with passion? One of the most beautiful examples I have encountered of living a passionate life is Bronwen Healy. I first met her through my editor at Regal. He told me, "You have got to meet this amazing woman, Bronwen, a former prostitute and drug addict, who is now the CEO of HOPE Foundation." So I called her on the telly (she's from Australia) and we hit it off instantly. I can tell you she is truly amazing. The HOPE Foundation, also based in Australia, exists "to bring liberty to sex workers and addicts through consistent Christ-centered connection and care," and they are doing just that every single day.

Some of the ways God allows HOPE to do this is through acts of service to women who work in the sex industry, who Bronwen refers to as "future lights to the world." On Valentine's Day and "Christmas in July," these incredible women and their children are blessed, pampered, fed, loved, prayed for and told over and over again in many different ways that they are loved and valued and created with a purpose! A dedicated team of more than 50 volunteers demonstrates this truth through flowers, jewelry, cards, chocolates, amazing food and desserts, and pampering treatments such as manicures, pedicures and massages. These women also are given the opportunity to express themselves through art, jewelry making and photography. During HOPE Foundation events, words of love, life and value are sown into the women, some of whom have *never* heard such truth before.

One at a time, God transforms the lives of women through the power of love and through the HOPE team's willingness to speak truth without being ashamed of the power of the gospel. The women can decide to leave their contact information and become one of a growing number of women seeking one-on-one mentoring. In that process, HOPE Foundation sees many women loved to wholeness and then become priceless benefits to their community. Every word is a seed, and the fruit is phenomenal!

Bronwen is proof that God can give you beauty for ashes and turn your pain into passionate service to others in His name. Bronwen says it best: "I know that the best way to feel elegant and precious in His sight is to give to others what has been given to me—truth, worth, value, forgiveness and freedom—from Jesus, but through others."[5]

## ONE LAST THOUGHT

If you start to get impatient, remember that living the life God designed for you is a process. This passage from the cherished children's book *The Velveteen Rabbit* by Margery Williams Bianco reflects the beauty and struggle of the journey. In the story, two toys, the Skin Horse and the Rabbit, talk about becoming Real:

> "Does it hurt?" asked the Rabbit.
> "Sometimes," said the Skin Horse, for he was always truthful.
> "When you are Real, you don't mind being hurt."

"Does it happen all at once, like being wound up," he asked, "or bit by bit?"

"It doesn't happen all at once," said the Skin Horse. "You become. It takes a long time. That's why it doesn't often happen to people who break easily, or have sharp edges, or who have to be carefully kept. Generally, by the time you are Real, most of your hair has been loved off, and your eyes drop out and you get loose in the joints and very shabby. But these things don't matter at all, because once you are Real you can't be ugly, except to people who don't understand."[6]

As you discover your passion pathway, remember Real dreams, Real service and Real passion are signature marks of a truly beautiful life.

## INTERVIEW WITH JOHN TESH: PASSION AND PRAYER

One of the exercises I talk about is to ask five important people in your life to tell you what they see you doing. That doesn't mean five people in your current life. Track down your creative writing or history teacher in high school. Or an old buddy from college or pastor. Just try to find people from different parts of your life and say, "Listen, I'm trying to figure out what I need to be doing. You probably know what I'm doing for a living, but I want to go where my heart is. Can you tell me what you have always seen me doing?" I did this and nobody said they saw me being on television. In fact, they all said they saw me sitting behind a grand piano playing with an orchestra because everyone knew that was my passion. . . .

The three big ways to get there—and these are in the book— are hard work, risk and prayer. You can't get anywhere without hard work. Getting there is never some sort of accident. The risk is a big one because risk implies that you have to be absent of fear. So many of us end up doubting what we are supposed to risk. In many studies of 90-year-olds, where they have been asked what they would have changed in their lives, they said they would risk more.

*Prayer* is essential. If you can't focus, you can't stay the course without having that connection with God. So the hard work, risk and prayer method works for me. Also learn to focus and simplify. Tell everyone you know what you want to do. Say, "I want to be a concert pianist with an orchestra." Speak as though you are that person, and then the people around you will start asking you, "Did you practice today? Did you connect today with someone who has a record deal? What are you doing to keep you on that course?" And eventually, on some level, that will be so.[7]

*My Passionate Daughter,*

Remember, you live and exist *in Me*. I'm your very being! Even before you were born, I destined you for purpose! *You are My* workmanship created in Jesus to do good works that I've already prepared *in advance* for you to accomplish. I'm making your life beautiful in My time. *Rejoice* and do good. Keep in mind that your face reflects My glory! Even when you don't realize it, I'm transforming you into My likeness with an *ever-increasing* glory. I'm at work in you to will and to act according to My good purpose. *Avoid* complaining and arguing. Instead, let Me make you *pure and* blameless. I'll help the *beauty* of your life to shine to others.

Unfolding your beauty,

*Your Creator*

Acts 17:28; Psalm 139:16; Ephesians 2:10; Ecclesiastes 3:11-12; 2 Corinthians 3:18

(By LeAnn Weiss-Rupard)

# Fourteen

# Bonus: Helping Your Man Look Grand

Orlando Magic Senior VP Pat Williams wears eye crème and loves it. Musician John Tesh, entrepreneur and motivator Peter Lowe and pastor Robert Schuller, Jr., know how to stock a pantry and eat healthy. Olympic gold medalist Josh Davis knows what it takes to be a "gold-medal man." All these guys have style and spirit, and your husband can, too!

I'm willing to bet that your man, while he may read leadership books or adventure novels, won't pick up a book on how to dress or how to care for his skin, unless he's a metro man. You can build your man's confidence without making him feel like a loser. Gently help him discover how to maximize his appearance—from skin to hair to clothing—in a way that makes him feel successful and huggable (and good-smelling, too!).

Women are not the only ones out there who care about what they look like, right? Men have mirrors,

> The whole idea of motivation is a trap. Forget motivation. Just do it. Exercise, lose weight, test your blood sugar, or whatever. Do it without motivation. And then, guess what? After you start doing the thing, that's when the motivation comes and makes it easy for you to keep on doing it.
>
> —John Maxwell

too—they just don't verbalize how much their appearance matters as often as women do. And so, to help your man feel his very best, here are some BBG tips on what to do, what to use and how to use it (mostly in bullet points to be guy-friendly!).

## BASIC GROOMING GUIDE

### Skincare: First Things First

What is your skin type? Meaning; are you "oily," "dry," "sensitive" or "normal"? Here's a quick way to find out:

- Wash your face with tepid water.

- Wait one hour. Is your face feeling dry or slick?

- Use a lens or blotting tissue to press around your face (forehead, nose, cheeks and chin). If the tissue comes away dry and your pores appear small, then your skin does not produce very much sebum (oil); this means that your skin type is dry. If the tissue comes away oily and your pores appear larger, your skin produces more sebum; this means that your skin type is oily. If your face is oily only in the T-zone (forehead, nose and chin) and dry or normal everywhere else, you likely have combination skin. If you have medium-sized pores with smooth skin tone, your skin type is considered *normal*.

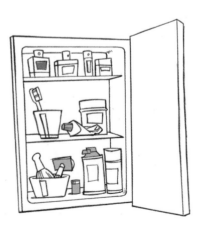

### Skincare Products

#### Normal to Dry Skin

- **Cleanser.** Aubrey Organics® Men's Stock Basic Cleansing Bar (www.aubrey-organics.com) has a low-scent facial bar made with 85 percent organic ingredients that leaves skin clean and refreshed without over-drying. You can use it in the shower.

Terressentials® (www.terresentials.com) makes a great kit called the Flower Therapy Skincare Sampler that has a cleanser, toner, lotion and crème (don't let the name fool you; it's "flower therapy" because hibiscus is a fantastic natural skin treatment).

- **Moisturizer.** Aubrey Organics Men's Stock Daily Moisturizer

## Oily Skin

- **Cleanser.** Mychelle® White Cranberry Cleanser cleans skin without over-drying, is 100-percent pure and smells invigorating (www.mychelleusa.com). The Organic Eucalyptus Seafoam Facial Cleanser made by 100% Pure® is also great for acne-prone skin (www.100percentpure.com).

- **Moisturizer.** MiEssence® Organics Purifying Moisturizer (www.miessence.com)

- **Blemish control.** Herbal Blemish Stick by Burt's Bees is excellent (www.burtsbees.com), or try tea tree oil.

## Sensitive Skin

- **Cleanser**. Unscented Cleansing Cream by CWS is a good option (www.allnaturalcosmetics.com). John Masters™ Organics Linden Blossom Face Cream Cleanser is gentle yet effective for sensitive skin (www.johnmasters.com).

- **Moisturizer.** Vegecol with Aloe Moisturizing Cream by Aubrey Organics

- **Treatment for dilated capillaries.** Capillary Calming Serum by Mychelle is a little pricey, but it works.

---

### Homemade Capillary Calmer

1 tablespoon jojoba oil
1 teaspoon macadamia oil
2 teaspoons sunflower oil
5 drops each German chamomile, calendula ($CO_2$ extract), helichrysum, lavender

*Mix all ingredients and let stand for 24 hours. Shake before each use and apply morning and night.[1] (For ingredients, check out www.mountainroseherbs.com.)*

### Toner

You can always make your own with Apple Cider Vinegar (dilute with water; not recommended for sensitive skin). Just apply to a cotton ball and dab on your face. Or buy Fruit Enzyme Mist by Mychelle (for all skin types) or 100% Pure's Organic Lavender Hydrosol or Peppermint Green Tea Refresher (most skin types, though eczema sometimes reacts to peppermint).

### Shave Cream

Try Avalon Organics Moisturizing Cream Shave, Organic Grooming Shave Cream by Herban Cowboy® (www.vitasprings.com) or Gaia® Made for Men™ Shave Gel (www.gaiaskinnaturals.com).

### Aftershave

Aubrey Organics Men's Stock in North Woods, Spice Island or City Rhythms, or Smooth by Mychelle will help with irritation and are light on the skin. Another one to try is by Burt's Bees called Natural Skin Care for Men After Shave.

Pre-shave product is usually made of oil (castor oil, olive oil with essential oils) that softens coarse beard hair so that it is easier to cut. You may like So Clean by Mychelle, which can also double as a cleanser.

## Daily Skincare Routine

- **Most skin types:** Cleanse, shave, tone, apply aftershave, moisturize and dab on eye crème (if you're in a hurry, skip the aftershave)

- **Oily skin:** Cleanse, shave, tone, apply aftershave and moisturize

- **Heavy beard:** Cleanse, pre-shave, shave, tone, apply aftershave, moisturize and apply a beard cleanser or softener

- **Ingrown hair:** Cleanse, scrub, pre-shave, shave, tone, spot-treat, apply aftershave and moisturize

## Evening Skincare Routine

Cleanse, tone, moisturize.

## Occasional Skincare Routine

- **Masks.** Use once or twice a week, depending on skin type. A clay mask draws out impurities while a mask with oats soothes the skin. Try John Masters French Green Clay & Green Tea Purifying Mask.

- **Exfoliate.** Once a week should be enough (some say two to three, but too much can irritate your skin). You can use baking soda mixed with water, or grind up 1/2 cup oats and add 1/4 cup powdered milk and 1 teaspoon of cornmeal (store mixture in airtight container). When you're ready to exfoliate, add enough water to make a paste. Massage onto skin, then rinse.

## Got Nicks?

Try the eShave Alum Block; it costs about $15, but alum has hemostatic properties and stops bleeding quickly. Un-Petroleum Jelly by Alba Botanicals is a good choice, too.

## All-in-One

The Clenzology® Advanced Hygiene System by Garden of Life (www.vitaminshoppe.com) includes A.M. and P.M. cleansers (that purify not only your skin but also mucus membranes and nasal cavity), hand and body wash, tooth and gum solution, ear solution (to reduce buildup of excess wax) and a natural sea sponge. I bought it for my husband and found myself using it, too.

## Sun Protection

Use daily, preferably SPF-25 or higher. Also, wear a hat and sunglasses. Be sure to get checked out by a dermatologist yearly (all the guys I interviewed could not stress this enough).

## Eye Crèmes

Eye crèmes are highly concentrated and specially formulated to be multitaskers, addressing fine lines, wrinkles, dark circles and puffiness. A good eye crème should be part of any anti-aging protocol, applied before you put on your all-over moisturizer.

Use your ring finger when applying eye crème, as it is the weakest finger and won't apply as much pressure as others. This is a delicate area that should not be dragged or pulled; try "dotting" your eye crème instead of rubbing, to minimize pulling on the skin. Try Aubrey Organics Men's Stock Daily Rejuvenating Eye Cream, John Masters Organics Firming Eye Gel or 100% Pure Coffee Bean Eye Cream.

## Hair Care Products

- **For thinning hair:** Lamas Botanicals Chinese Herb Stimulating Shampoo works well (www.lamasbeauty.com). The Morrocco Method has a good system for hair growth and Desert Essence® Organics Thickening Shampoo (and Conditioner, too) Green Apple & Ginger has gotten good reviews (www.desertessence.com).

- **For normal to dry hair:** Burt's Bees Super Shiny Grapefruit & Sugar Beet shampoo is an affordable choice, while John Masters Organics and Dessert Essences are both very effective for dry scalp.

- **Styling gels:** Try Aubrey Organics Men's Stock Ginseng Biotin Hair Gel, MiEssence Organic Shape Styling Gel or the Scalp Rescue™ Gel or Pomade made by Max Green Alchemy® (www.maxgreenalchemy.com).

**BBG TIP**

When trimming eyebrows, cut in layers so that hairs don't stick straight out. If brows are unruly, apply castor oil with a Q-tip (be careful of eyes) to soften them.

## The Man in the Mirror

Before leaving the house, do the NENE-Check to make sure that no hair is left behind:

- Nose hair (trim)
- Ear hair (trim)
- Neck hair (shave)
- Eyebrow hair (trim)

## Smelling Good

Now that you have done the mirror check, you are ready for some cologne. Why not try an alternative fragrance brand that does not contain phthalates or parabens, such as Pacifica (www.pacificaperfume.com). Pacifica is a family-owned company out of Oregon that has a wonderful line of lotions, soaps, candles and fragrance. Some of my favorite scents are the Mediterranean Fig and Spanish Amber. (I am not a big fragrance person, but these smell great for guys and are very affordable.)

# CLOSET INTERVENTION

Your man likely has good taste in food—and obviously has great taste in women—but he may need some confidence-building when it comes to his taste in wardrobe. I watched the first man in my life, my dad (who worked in an upscale men's suit shop), dress and tailor men to their specific needs. Take your cue from Dad and help your honey look sharp.

Let's head to your husband's closet. If an article of clothing has not been worn in two years, toss it, along with any "I'll wear it when I lose 10 pounds" items. (His intentions are good, but the reality is that it probably won't happen overnight.)

What should be in his closet, his Essentials for Potential? He should have at least:

- A two- or three-button tropical-weight wool suit in black, charcoal gray or navy
- A sport coat
- Six dress shirts (sized to neck and sleeve) in a variety of colors
- Six sports shirts (like Polos), long and/or short sleeve
- Six ties
- Three sweaters (spoil him with one in cashmere)

- An overcoat
- One pair each of brown loafers, black loafers and black lace-ups
- Two pairs of jeans, one in a medium wash for weekends, and one dark
- One pair of cargo, painter or carpenter pants
- A brown belt and a black belt
- A leather briefcase

## IN THEIR OWN WORDS

I asked some guys about taking care of themselves. Here's what they said:

### On Style

> I have turned [style] over to my wife. . . . She was in charge of the lighting for the show [his live DVD, *Alive*] . . . she is also in charge of how I dress.
> —*John Tesh*

> Men's Warehouse has a great affordable selection. I suit up for speaking engagements, but otherwise I wear a Hawaiian shirt.
> —*Pat Williams*

> My wife picks out my clothes, except for my daily outfit, a bathing suit.
> —*Josh Davis*

### On Health

> I have tried everything and I'm all about knowing your limitations. For example, I know that I tend to overeat when I go out to dinner. My wife is not an overeater, so she works with me on this. So when we go out, we might order an entree and split it, or just order appetizers, not a main course.
>
> Portion control is a really big deal. Never eat mindlessly. Never eat in front of the television, never eat while you're standing up.

Try to never eat at your desk. Mindful eating means you'll eat a lot less food.

I have found a [trainer] that works with me. He and I agreed on a set dollar amount every month, whether I show up or not, and I don't get a refund. Every morning he shows up at 6 A.M. and I'd better be out of bed. . . . We box, we jump rope, we do pushups together. It's an appointment. I don't wake up saying I hope I get to work out today. It's the first thing I do every day. It's the only way I can stay stable.
—*John Tesh*

I wake up every morning and grab a bowl of whole-grain cereal with fruit or oatmeal. Then I work out for an hour swimming every day.
—*Josh Davis*

I pick up five newspapers, read them and eat cold cereal. I work out with weights and do cardio every day. I just ran my forty-ninth marathon this past April; it was actually my twelfth Boston Marathon. We are all getting in shape for old age. [After visiting his mother in a nursing home, Pat said] If you have any doubts about working out, that should inspire you. The body was made to exercise; the man sitting on the couch is living dangerously.
—*Pat Williams*

## Personal Growth

Intentional growth is essential for your success in marriage, relationships, work and daily living. Here are a few choices for your library:

- *Intelligence for Your Life: Powerful Lessons for Personal Growth* by John Tesh (Nashville, TN: Thomas Nelson, 2008). I read it and gave it to my husband, who also loved it.

- *Destination Success: A Map for Living Out Your Dreams* by Dwight Bain (Grand Rapids, MI: Revell, 2003). Find direction and purpose, gain confidence and break free from self-destructive patterns.

- *The Goal and the Glory: Christian Athletes Share Their Inspiring Stories* by Josh Davis (Ventura, CA: Regal, 2008). More than 30 Olympians share life lessons and personal moments to inspire you to set goals for yourself.

- *The Pursuit: Wisdom for the Adventure of Your Life* by Pat Williams (Ventura, CA: Regal, 2008). Pat has written many books, but here he shares six practical insights that are essential for success in life.

- *Perfect Weight America: Change Your Diet, Change Your Life, Change Your World* by Jordan Rubin (Orlando, FL: Siloam Press, 2008) is a fabulous read, with beneficial information about health, fitness and tasty recipes.

# *Beauty by God*

## Resources

✢ ✢ ✢

## PERSONAL CARE

### Acne Treatment

*Skinnutrients Accunatural* www.skinutrients.com (do not use if you are allergic to strawberries)

### Beauty Supplements

*Bio Nativus Inner Beauty* www.bionativus.com

*Rejuva* www.rejuvarx.com

### Breast Health

*Nature's Way DIM-plus* (one of my pastors' wives swears by this, not just for breast health but for hormonal issues as well) www.myvitanet.com

*NewMark Zyflamend* www.new-mark.com

### Detox*

*Dr. Natura* (Toxin-Out and Colonix) www.drnatura.com

*Healing Herbal Soups* www.healingherbalsoups.com

*RenewLife CleanseSMART* (First Cleanse two-week program) www.vitacost.com

### Essential Oils

*Mountain Rose Herbs* www.mountainroseherbs.com

*Wyndmere Essential Oils* www.whole-food-vitamins.net

*Young Living* www.youngliving.us

---

*\* Be sure to check with your doctor before attempting any cleanse.*

## Feminine Products

*Natracare* www.natracare.com

*Seventh Generation* www.seventhgeneration.com

## Fitness

*Rebounding* www.reboundair.com

*Stott Pilates* www.stottpilates.com

*T-Tapp* www.t-tapp.com

*Yamuna Body Rolling* www.yamunabodyrolling.com

## Hair Care

*Color* Herbatint or Naturtint www.ihealthtree.com, Tints of Nature
www.tintsofnatureusa.com

*Gels and pomades* Aubrey Organics, Max Green Alchemy
www.maxgreenalchemy.com

*Growth* Alphactif www.drugstore.com, Hair Genesis www.hairgenesis.net,
The Morrocco Method www.morroccomethod.com

*Shampoo and conditioner* Desert Essence, John Masters Organics

*Spray* AVEDA www.aveda.com, Privè www.priveproducts.com, Suncoat
www.suncoatproducts.com (both Privè and AVEDA contain
some synthetic ingredients)

*Salons* If you are in the Orlando, Florida, area, please visit Salon Salon
and ask for Lulu, or contact her at luluandherhair@hotmail.com.
Also visit Celia Hoyo at Main Street Tanning Salon and Spa the
next time you are in Orlando (www.mainstreettansalon.com).

## Hygiene

*Deodorant* Aubrey Organics, Dr. Hauschka, Young Living Oils, Herbal
Magic www.vitamincountry.com

*Toothpaste* A Wild Soap Bar Tooth Savior tooth soap
www.awildsoapbar.com

## Makeup

*100% Pure* www.100percentpure.com (also on QVC)

*AfterGlow* www.afterglowcosmetics.com

*Alima* www.alimapure.com

*Beauty Blender* (applicator) www.beautyblender.net

*Dr. Hauschka* www.drhauschka.com
*Jane Iredale* www.janeiredaledirect.com
*Lavera* www.lavera.com
*Living Nature* www.livingnature.com
*MiEssence* www.elyorganics.com
*Monavé* www.monave.com
*Suki* www.sukipure.com
*ZuZu Luxe* www.gabrielcosmetics.com

## Nail Polish and Removers

*Honeybee Gardens* www.honeybeegardens.com
*No-Miss* www.nomiss.com
*SpaRitual* www.sparitual.com
*Suncoat* www.suncoatproducts.com
*Zoya* www.zoya.com

## Perfume

*Aubrey Organics* www.aubrey-organics.com
*JoAnne Bassett* www.joannebassett.com
*Kuumba Made* www.kuumbamade.com
*Le Labo* www.lelabofragrances.com
*Mandy Aftel* www.aftlier.com
*Pacifica Perfumes* www.pacificacandles.com
*Puresha* www.puresha.com
*Wyndmere Essential Oils* www.wyndmerenaturals.com

## Skin Care

*100% Pure* www.100percentpure.com
*Aubrey Organics* www.aubrey-organics.com
*Blooming Lotus* www.bloominglotus.com
*Burt's Bees* www.burtsbees.com
*Coconut Clean* www.coconutclean.com
*Dr. Hauschka* www.drhauschka.com
*John Masters Organics* www.johnmasters.com
*Jurlique* www.jurlique.com

*MiEssence* www.elyorganics.com
*Mychelle* www.mychelleusa.com
*Naturopathica* www.naturopathica.com
*Osmosis Pur Medical Skin Care* www.osmosisskincare.com
*Pangea Organics* www.pangeaorganics.com
*Spa Technologies* www.spatechnologies.com

## Supplements

*Green foods* Garden of Life www.gardenoflife.com, New Chapter Berry
    Greens www.new-chapter.com
*Fish and cod liver oil* Olde World Icelandic Cod Liver Oil made by
    Garden of Life, Carlson Lemon Flavor Cod Liver Oil
    www.carlsonlabs.com
*Probiotic* Primal Defense Ultra made by Garden of Life
    www.gardenoflifeusa.com
*Vitamins/nutrients* Garden of Life, New Chapter, www.vibe.com,
    www.prlabs.com

# HOME CARE

## Bathroom

*Shower curtain* (hemp) www.healthfoodstore.com
*Bathmat* www.alsoto.com, www.realgoods.com
*Towels* Gaiam www.gaiam.com, Target www.target.com

## Beverages

*Numi tea* www.ihealthtree.com
*Pure Inventions* www.pureinventions.com
*Teeccino Mediterranean and Mayan herbal coffees* www.teeccino.com
*Tulsi teas* www.omorganics.com

## Candles

*Blue Corn Naturals* www.beeswaxcandles.com
*Pacifica Candles* www.pacificacandles.com
*Scandle* (melts into body lotion) www.abodycandle.com

## Clean Air

*Air purifier* PCI-AIRE www.bioactivenutrients.com, UV air purifier
www.realgoods.com
*Salt lamp* www.thesaltoftheearth.com
*Water purifier* www.newwaveenviro.com

## Cleaning Supplies

*Bio-Kleen* www.biokleen.com
*Seventh Generation*

## House Plants (to purify your air!)

Areca palm
Bamboo plant
Boston fern
English ivy
Dracaena "Janet Craig"
Dwarf date palm
Ficus alii
Lady palm
Peace lily
Rubber plant

## Spices and Salts

*Organic spices and seasoning packets* www.spicehunter.com
*Premier Pink Salt* www.prlabs.com

## Sweeteners

*Xylitol* www.xlearinc.com
Also try agave nectar, lua han guo and honey

# *Endnotes*

## Chapter 1: God's View of Beauty and Balance

1. Dove Global Study: The Truth about Beauty, at the Dove Campaign for Real Beauty. www.campaignforrealbeauty.com/supports.asp?id=92&length=short&section= campaign&src=InsideCampaign_globalstudy (accessed January 2007). These figures and other similar statistics are part of the Real Truth About Beauty study, compiled by the Campaign for Real Beauty, a Dove-sponsored global survey of 3,200 girls and women between the ages of 18 and 64, from the United States to Saudi Arabia. The campaign is designed to open a debate on body image and beauty stereotypes through education, online forums, a self-esteem fund and inspirational stories.

2. Ibid.

3. "About BodyImageHealth.org," BodyImageHealth.org. http://www.bodyimagehealth.org/about.html (accessed January 2007).

4. Bobby and Peter Farrelly, *Shallow Hal*, "Quotes," IMDb: Earth's Biggest Movie Database. http://www.imdb.com/title/tt0256380/quotes (accessed January 2007).

5. The Body Shop International, 1997 campaign. http://www.thebodyshopinternational.com/Values+and+Campaigns/Our+Campaigns/ (accessed January 2007).

6. Activity Sheet 2.4 courtesy of the Dove Campaign for Real Beauty. http://www.campaignforrealbeauty.co.uk/dsef/pdfs/BodyTalk_Excerpt.pdf, (accessed January 2007).

7. Dr. Susie Orbach, Activity Sheet 2.2 courtesy of the Dove Campaign for Real Beauty (accessed January 2007).

8. British Medical Association, Activity Sheet 2.2 courtesy of the Dove Campaign for Real Beauty (accessed January 2007).

9. Alex Kuczynski, *Beauty Junkies: Inside Our $15 Billion Obsession with Cosmetic Surgery* (New York: Doubleday, 2006), cover copy.

10. "The Foot Facelift: Cosmetic Surgery for Your Feet," Surgerynews.net. http://surgery news.net/news/111003/other007.html (accessed January 2007).

11. "Foot Cosmetic Surgery Catching On," CBS Broadcasting, Inc., May 20, 2005. http://www.cbsnews.com/stories/2005/05/20/earlyshow/health/main696806.shtml (accessed January 2007).

12. "Plastic Surgery Complications Killed Woman," at IrishHealth.com. http://www.irish health.com/?level=4&id=7603 (accessed July 2008).

13. David C. Pack, "The Truth Hidden Behind Makeup," Restored Church of God, http://www.thercg.org/books/tthbm.html (accessed July 2008).

14. "Cosmetics," Wikipedia, http://en.wikipedia.org/wiki/Cosmetics (accessed January 2007).

15. Pack, "The Truth Hidden Behind Makeup."

16. Ibid.

17. Quoted in Rob Bell, *Sex God: Exploring the Endless Connections Between Sexuality and Spirituality* (Grand Rapids, MI: Zondervan, 2007).

18. Marlie Casseus, as told to Jacqueline Charles, "Real Life: 'I had a 21-pound Tumor on My Face,'" *Seventeen*, January 2007, p. 60.

## Chapter 2: Get Glowing, Gorgeous and Green

1. Jordan Rubin, author of *Perfect Weight America: Change Your Diet, Change Your Life, Change Your World* (Lake Mary, FL: Siloam Press, 2008), in an interview with the author, April 2008.

2. Sharad Teheri, Ling Lin, Diane Austin, Terry Young and Emmanuel Mignot, "Short Sleep Duration Is Associated with Reduced Leptin, Elevated Ghrelin, and Increased Body Mass Index," Public Library of Science (Medicine), December 2004. http://www.pubmed central.nih.gov/articlerender.fcgi?artid=535701 (accessed September 2008).

3. For more information on ERVs, visit www.greenbuilder.com/sourcebook/Energy RecoveryVent.html#Consider.

4. Tom Watson, "Coated Pots and Pans Can Present Health Hazards," *Seattle Times,* August 10, 2007, posted by Environmental Working Group, http://www.ewg.org/node/22396 (accessed June 2008).

5. Compiled from www.truthinlabeling.org (accessed May 2008).

6. Susan Swithers, as quoted by Amy Patterson-Neubert, "Study: Artificial Sweetener May Disrupt Body's Ability to Count Calories," *Purdue News*, June 29, 2004, http://news.uns.purdue.edu/html4ever/2004/040629.Swithers.research.html (accessed August 2008).

7. You can find out more about labeling from *Consumer Reports'* Greener Choices Eco-Label Center, http://www.greenerchoices.org/ (accessed August 2008).

9. Luddene Perry and Dan Schultz, *A Field Guide to Buying Organic* (New York: Bantam Books, 2005).

10. "Shopper's Guide to Pesticides in Produce," Food News from the Environmental Working Group, http://www.foodnews.org/walletguide.php (accessed August 2008).

11. Lynn Schultz, cofounder of 1-800-HEALTHY, in an interview with the author, March 2008.

12. Jordan Rubin interview, April 2008.

13. Information regarding detoxification compiled from gloriagilbere.com, jointcare101.com, http://www.naturalhealingtoday.com/detox_and_diet.html, http://www.drnatura.com/?gclid=CMnO5aXNq5ACFUaPOAodqSD0NA, and Robert O. Young, and Shelley Redford Young , *The pH Miracle: Balance Your Diet, Reclaim Your Health* (New York: Warner Books, 2002).

14. Rubin, *Perfect Weight America*, p. 30.

15. Ibid., p. 67.

16. Ibid., p. 132.

17. Carl Zimmer, "Do Parasites Rule the World?" *Discover* magazine, August 2000. http://find articles.com/p/articles/mi_m1511/is_8_21/ai_63583791/pg_1 (accessed September 2008).

18. *Body Story: Body Snatchers*, © Discovery Communications, Inc.

19. Dr. Gloria Gilbére, author of *I Was Poisoned by My Body* (Lancaster, OH: Lucky Press, 2000), in an interview with the author, March 2008.

20. Ibid.

21. Young and Young , *The pH Miracle*, p. 277.

22. Dr. Gloria Gilbére interview, March 2008.

23. Ibid.

24. Al Carter, founder of ReboundAIR, Inc., in an interview with the author, April 2008.

## Chapter 3: Beauty 101: Skincare

1. Ben Johnson, CEO, Osmosis Skincare, in an interview with the author, January 2008.

2. Amy Larocca, "Liquid Gold in Morocco," *New York Times* online, *T* Magazine: Travel, November 18, 2007. http://travel.nytimes.com/2007/11/18/travel/tmagazine/14get-sourcing-caps.html (accessed June 2008).

3. Doris J. Day and Sandra Forsyth, *Forget the Face Lift: Turn Back the Clock with a Revolutionary Program for Ageless Skin* (New York: Penguin Books, 2005), p. 92.

4. Denise Blair, Dermal Institute, in an interview with the author, February 2008.

5. Ruth Winter, MS, *A Consumer's Dictionary of Cosmetic Ingredients* (New York: Three Rivers Press, 2005), p. 315.

6. Denise Blair interview, February 2008.

7. Ibid.

8. Peter C. Pacik, MD, FACS, "Sun Damage/Sun Protection," SkinCare-MD.com Articles. http://www.skincare-md.com/index.cfm?event=showStory&storyid=15 (accessed September 2008).

9. Denise Blair interview, February 13, 2008.

10. Information regarding product expiration dates compiled from "Tips for Safekeeping and Use of Cosmetics," Medical College of Wisconsin. http://www.healthlink.mcw.edu/article/975513403.html (accessed February 2008) and U.S. Food and Drug Administration Center for Food Safety and Applied Nutrition: Cosmetics. http://www.cfsan.fda.gov/~dms/cos-toc.html (accessed August 2008).

## Chapter 4: Face Forward: Steps to a Flawless Face

1. Eve Pearl, award-winning makeup artist, in an interview with the author, May 2007.

2. Marvin Westmore, founder of Westmore Academy, in an interview with the author, March 2007.

3. Ibid.

4. "Lipstick" at Wikipedia.org. http://en.wikipedia.org/wiki/Lipstick (accessed August 2008).

## Chapter 5: Haute, Healthy Hair

1. Christopher Hopkins, *Staging Your Comeback: A Complete Beauty Revival for Women Over 45* (Deerfield Beach, FL: HCI Books, 2008), p. 153.

## Chapter 6: The Devil's Top-10 Ingredients

1. David Steinman and Samuel S. Epstein, M.D., *The Safe Shopper's Bible: A Consumer's Guide to Nontoxic Household Products, Cosmetics, and Food* (New York: Wiley Publishing, 1995), p. 17.

2. Charlotte Vohtz, founder of Green People Company, http://www.telegraph.co.uk/health/main.jhtml?xml=/health/2005/03/18/hmake18.xml&page=1

3. The Environmental Working Group, "How Dangerous Are Your Cosmetics?" Skin Deep Executive Summary, Mercola.com, July 17, 2004. http://articles.mercola.com/sites/articles/archive/2004/07/17/dangerous-cosmetics.aspx (accessed September 2008).

4. "Risks of Talcum Powder," from the Cancer Prevention Coalition, Avoidable Exposures for Consumers. http://www.preventcancer.com/consumers/cosmetics/talc.htm (accessed June 2008).

5. "Coming Clean: Campaigning for Organic Integrity in Bodycare Products," Coming Clean Campaign, Organic Consumers Association. http://www.organicconsumers.org/bodycare/index.cfm (accessed August 2008).

6. See Darbre, Aljarrah, Miller, Coldham, Sauer and Pope, "Concentrations of Parabens in Human Breast Tumours, *Journal of Applied Toxicology*, Jan.-Feb. 2004, and SCCP, "Opinion on Parabens. Colipa," No. P82, 10 Oct 2006.

7. Dr. Gloria Gilbére interview, March 2008.

8. "Triclosan: Health Concerns" at Wikipedia.org. http://en.wikipedia.org/wiki/Triclosan#Health_concerns (accessed September 2008). See also "Plain Soap as Effective as Antibacterial but Without the Risk," Physorg.com, August 15, 2007. http://www.physorg.com/news106418144.html (accessed September 2008).

9. Christine Hoza Farlow, *Dying to Look Good: The Disturbing Truth about What's Really in Your Cosmetics, Toiletries and Personal Care Products* (Escondido, CA: KISS for Health Publishing, 2005), p. 33.

10. "Scientific Facts on Phthalates," from GreenFacts: Facts on Health and the Environment, GreenFacts.org. http://www.greenfacts.org/phthalates/index.htm (accessed June 2008).

11. Jane Kay, "Toxic Toys," *San Francisco Chronicle*, Nov. 19, 2006. http://www.sfgate.com/cgi-bin/article.cgi?f=/c/a/2006/11/19/TOXICTOYS.TMP (accessed September 2008). See also Environmental Working Group, "Research: Why This Matters" at the Cosmetic

Safety Database online. http://www.cosmeticsdatabase.com/research/whythismatters. php?nothanks=1 (accessed September 2008).

12. Material Safety Data Sheet: Triethanolamine MSDS. http://www.sciencelab.com/ xMSDS-Triethanolamine-9927306 (accessed August 2008).

13. Stacy Malkan, *Not Just A Pretty Face: The Ugly Side of the Beauty Industry* (Gabriola Island, B.C., Canada: New Society Publishers, 2007), p. 17.

14. Ibid., pp. 72,74.

15. Narelle Chenery, director of research and development for Miessence® Certified Organic Skin, Hair, Body and Health Products, in an interview with the author, August 2008.

16. Ibid.

17. Ruth Winter, *A Consumer's Dictionary of Cosmetic Ingredients: Complete Information About the Harmful and Desirable Ingredients Found in Cosmetics and Cosmeceuticals* (New York: Three Rivers Press), p. 469.

18. "About Us," Restoring Eden: Christians for Environmental Stewardship. http://www.restoring eden.org/about (accessed August 2008).

19. "Campaigns," Restoring Eden: Christian for Environment Stewardship. www.restoring eden.org/campaigns (accessed June 2008).

## Chapter 8: Clothing Essentials for Potential

1. Brenda Kinsel, *Brenda Kinsel's Fashion Makeover: 30 Days to Diva Style!* (San Francisco: Chronicle Books, 2007), p. 69.

2. Allison Houte interview, March 2008.

3. "Numbers to Know," Harper's Bazaar Fakes Are Never in Fashion Campaign. http://fakes areneverinfashion.com/fakes_numbers.asp (accessed August 2008).

4. Adapted from Shelly Ballestero, "The J-Factor," *On Course* magazine, March 10, 2008. http:// oncourse.ag.org/features/index.cfm?targetBay=06d52a80-8681-49b2-871b-a4e5dc1c 7708&ModID=2&Process=DisplayArticle&RSS_RSSContentID=6067&RSS_OriginatingChan nelID=1202&RSS_OriginatingRSSFeedID=3459&RSS_Source= (accessed August 2008).

5. Shaunti Feldhahn, *For Women Only: What You Need to Know About the Inner Lives of Men* (Sisters, OR: Multnomah, 2004).

6. Danielle Kimmey interview, April 2008.

7. Adapted from "How to Hold a Fashion Swap Party," at WikiHow.com. http://www.wiki how.com/Hold-a-Fashion-Swap-Party (accessed August 2008).

## Chapter 9: Luxury Living for Less

1. Sharon Durling, *A Girl and Her Money* (Nashville, TN: Thomas Nelson, 2003), p. 52.

2. John Tesh, "Save Money on Your Next Family Vacation," Tesh.com. http://www.tesh.com/ ittrium/visit?path=A1xc797x1y1xa5x1x76y1x2413x1x9by1x2418x1y5x466fx5x1 (accessed August 2008).

3. Adapted from Jennifer "Gin" Sanders, *Wear More Cashmere: 151 Luxurious Ways to Pamper Your Inner Princess* (Beverly, MA: Fair Winds Press, 2003).

## Chapter 10: Scents and Sensibilities

1. Cathy Newman, *Perfume: The Art and Science of Scent* (Washington, DC: National Geographic Society Books, 1998), p. 67.

2. Stacy Malkan, *Not Just A Pretty Face: The Ugly Side of the Beauty Industry* (Gabriola Island, B.C., Canada: New Society Publishers, 2007), p. 59.

3. Ibid.

4. Mandy Aftel, founder of Aftelier Perfumes and author of *Essence & Alchemy: A Natural History of Perfume* (Layton, UT: Gibbs Smith, 2004), in an interview with the author, June 2008.

5. Ibid.

6. Athena Thompson, certified building biologist and author of *Homes that Heal (and Those that Don't): How Your Home Could Be Harming Your Family's Health* (Gabriola Island, B.C., Canada: New Society Publishers, 2004), in an interview with the author, April 2008.

7. Ibid.

## Chapter 11: Alleviate Stinkin' Thinkin'

1. David Stoop, *Self-Talk: Key to Personal Growth* (Grand Rapids: Revell, 1982), p. 65.

2. Ibid.

3. Ibid., p. 67.

4. Neil T. Anderson and David Park, *Overcoming Negative Self Image* (Ventura, CA: Regal Books, 2003), p. 74.

5. Joel Osteen, Audio Podcast #321: *Having Confidence in Yourself.*

6. Laurie Mintz, University of Missouri-Columbia, "Media Has Powerful Effect on Body Image Satisfaction," Aphrodite Women's Health, March 28, 2007. http://www.aphrodite womenshealth.com/news/20070228020255_health_news.shtml (accessed June 2008).

7. Ibid.

8. *USA Today*, August 12, 1996, 01D, via the National Institute on Media and the Family, "Media's Effect on Girls: Body Image and Gender Identity" online Fact Sheet. http://www.mediafamily.org/facts/facts_mediaeffect.shtml (accessed September 2008).

9. M. Tiggemann and A. S. Pickering, "Role of Television in Adolescent Women's Body Dissatisfaction and Drive for Thinness," *International Journal of Eating Disorders*, vol. 20 (1996), pp. 199-203.

10. Joan Jacobs Brumberg, *The Body Project: An Intimate History of American Girls* (New York: Random House, 1997), n.p.

11. D. Hargreaves, "Idealized Women in TV Ads Make Girls Feel Bad," *Journal of Social and Clinical Psychology*, 21 (2002), pp. 287-308.

12. Elizabeth Hurley, quoted by Imogene Tilden and Sara Gaines, "Marilyn Monroe," *The Guardian*, June 1, 2001. http://www.guardian.co.uk/news/2001/jun/01/netnotes.saragaines (accessed August 2008).

13. Amber Weigand-Buckley, "Conversation: Mandisa: My New Perspective," The Pentecostal Evangel, October 21, 2007. http://pentecostalevangel.ag.org/Conversations 2007/4876_Mandisa.cfm (accessed September 2008). Used by permission.

14. Scott Steindorff, quoted at Penelopethemovie.com, paraphrased by the author.

15. Lucie Costa, founder and editor of *Beautiful One* magazine, in an interview with the author, May 2008.

16. Darlene Schacht, *The Mom Complex* (Winnipeg, Manitoba, Canada: Spilt Milk Publishing, 2006), p. 84.

17. Linda Mintle, Ph.D., "I Think I Can, I Think I Can: Don't Let Negative Self-Talk Control Who You Are," *Joyce Meyer Magazine*, January 2008, pp. 21-22.

## Chapter 12: Jealousy: Beauty Turned Beast

1. Joyce Meyer, *Battlefield of the Mind: Winning the Battle in Your Mind* (New York: Hachette Book Group, 2002), pp. 263-264.

2. Michelle McKinney Hammond, video interview, iQuestions.com. http://www.iquestions.com/video/view/1037 (accessed June 2008).

3. Anita Renfroe, in an interview with the author, February 2008.

4. Kent Crockett, *I Once Was Blind, But Now I Squint* (Chattanooga, TN: AMG Publishers, 2004), p. 65.

5. Abigail Mason, in an interview with the author, February 2008.

6. Jennifer Rothschild, video interview, on iQuestions.com. http://www.iquestions.com/video/view/911 (accessed June 2008).

## Chapter 13: Discover Your Passion Pathway

1. Amber Buckley, in an interview with the author, December 2007.

2. John Avant, *The Passion Promise: Living a Life Only God Can Imagine* (Sisters, OR: Multnomah Books, 2004), n.p.

3. Susan Jeffers, PhD, *Feel the Fear and Do It Anyway* (New York: Ballantine Books, 2006).

4. CC, in an interview with the author, March 2008.

5. Bronwen Healy, in an interview with the author, March 2008.

6. Margery Williams, *The Velveteen Rabbit, or How Toys Become Real*, University of Pennsylvania Digital Library. http://digital.library.upenn.edu/women/williams/rabbit/rabbit.html (accessed August 2008).

7. John Tesh, in an interview with the author, April 2008.

## Chapter 14: Bonus: Helping Your Man Look Grand

1. Stephanie Tourles, *Organic Body Care Recipes* (North Adams, MA: Storey Publishing, 2007).

# Thanks to . . .

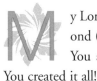

y Lord and Savior for the gifts of life, family, forgiveness, second (third, fourth . . . a ton of) chances, mercy and grace. You are beautiful; everything is "Beauty by God," because You created it all!

My loving husband, Angelo, who told me to keep going when I wanted to quit and who has loved me every step of the way. I am a better person because of you.

Angelo and Christopher, my beautiful and wonderful boys: You are mighty warriors of God.

My mom, Betty Choquette, who always supports me, and my mom's husband, Bob.

My sister, Lisa, who I love dearly.

LeAnn Weiss-Rupard, my best friend and spiritual sister. You are the ultimate encourager! You saw a book in me *way* before I ever did, and when I wanted to give up, you lifted me up. I am forever grateful!

Glenn Wagner, my agent, for helping me to stay focused.

Janis Whipple, my friend and editor: I would need another book to tell you how thankful I am for you!

Steve Lawson, who is a great editor and encourager. Without your perseverance, this book could not have happened; I owe you tons of Starbucks coffee!

Aly Hawkins, for your editorial expertise, and to Kirsten Van Peursem, Mark Weising, Rob Williams, Brenda Usery and the whole Regal team—you guys are great!

Maryellen and Dave Murray, who are gifts from God.

Amber Weigand-Buckley, who is so special, and to Amber's husband, Phil—you both are great!

Danika and Stephen Felts, who are both amazing.

Uncle (Dr.) Robert Forsely, for your wisdom.

Elle and Mike Brasell, who are great friends.

Virginia Ann Rodriquez and Jim and Mialena, for your support.

Kim Alexis, an inspiring woman of God, for being a part of this book. You are a "super model" for us all.

Lisa Mcintire, who is so talented. Thanks for your help!

Paulette and Mez Varol, for your generosity in allowing me to go to such a great school (The International Academy in South Daytona, Florida, owned by great people of God)!

Dan Gracey, for your talent.

Leslie Graham, my great friend, focus partner and prayer partner.

Sheila Viadero, my lifelong friend.

Doug and Coni Rhudy, for your support and friendship.

Rodger and Brenda Long, for having the best Christian bookstore around: Long's Christian Books and Music store!

Deana Spratt, my skincare partner and my wonderful friend.

Eve Pearl, who is beautiful inside and out.

Tamara Lowe, for sharing your wisdom. You are inspiring.

Darlene Schadt, for Christian Women Online; to Laura Bagby, my wonderful CBN.com Internet producer; and to Lucie Costa, of *Beautiful One* magazine.

Teresa Tapp, for your part in this book (oh, and for Kitty putting us together!).

Alison Houtte, Holly Wagner, Brenda Kinsel, Jane Iredale, Nicole C. Mullen, Tammy Trent, Mandisa, John Tesh, Denise Blair, Josh Davis, Pat Williams, Torry Martin, Jordan Rubin, Athena Thompson, Stacy Malkin, the Environmental Working Group, Bronwen Healey, Candace Cameron-Bure, Carla Williams, Billie Wilson, Grace Knodt, Ron Kenoly, Danielle Kimmey, Abigail Mason, Milette and Lee Brown, Al Carter, Marvin Westmore, John Masters, Barbara Close, Michelle McKinney, Anita Renfroe, Dr. Gloria Gilbère, Dr. Don Mayfield, Robert and Donna Schuller, Denise Blair, Dr. Ben Johnson, and Bryan Lenox (and your lovely wife, Tammy, and your boys) . . .

# More Great Resources from
# Regal Books

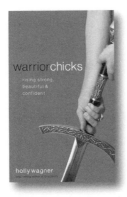
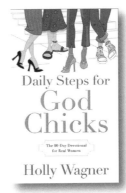
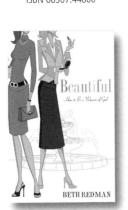
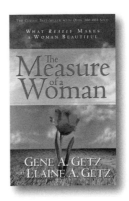
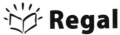